Complex Injuries of the Foot and Ankle in Sport

Guest Editor

DAVID A. PORTER, MD, PhD

FOOT AND ANKLE CLINICS

www.foot.theclinics.com

Consulting Editor
MARK S. MYERSON, MD

June 2009 • Volume 14 • Number 2

SAUNDERS an imprint of ELSEVIER, Inc.

W.B. SAUNDERS COMPANY
A Division of Elsevier Inc.

1600 John F. Kennedy Blvd. ● Suite 1800 ● Philadelphia, PA 19103-2899

http://www.theclinics.com

FOOT AND ANKLE CLINICS Volume 14, Number 2
June 2009 ISSN 1083-7515, ISBN-10: 1-4377-0476-X, ISBN-13: 978-1-4377-0476-1

Editor: Debora Dellapena

Foot and Ankle Clinics (ISSN 1083-7515) is published quarterly by Elsevier, Inc., 360 Park Avenue South, New York, NY 10010-1710. Months of issue are March, June, September, and December. Business and Editorial Offices: 1600 John F. Kennedy Blvd., Suite 1800, Philadelphia, PA 19103-2899. Customer Service Office: 11830 Westline Industrial Drive, St. Louis, MO 63146. Periodicals postage paid at New York, NY, and additional mailing offices. Subscription price per year is $230.00 (US individuals), $333.00 (US institutions), $116.00 (US students), $257.00 (Canadian individuals), $394.00 (Canadian institutions), $159.00 (Canadian students), $331.00 (foreign individuals), $394.00 (foreign institutions), and $159.00 (foreign students). To receive student/resident rate, orders must be accompanied by name of affiliated institution, date of term, and the *signature* of program/residency coordinator on institution letterhead. Orders will be billed at individual rate until proof of status is received. Foreign air speed delivery is included in all *Clinics* subscription prices. All prices are subject to change without notice. **POSTMASTER:** Send address changes to *Foot and Ankle Clinics*, Elsevier Periodicals Customer Service, 11830 Westline Industrial Drive, St. Louis, MO 63146. **Customer Service: 1-800-654-2452 (US). From outside of the United States, call 314-453-7041. Fax: 314-453-5170. E-mail: JournalsCustomerService-usa@elsevier.com (for print support); JournalsOnlineSupport-usa@elsevier. com (for online support).**

Reprints. For copies of 100 or more, of articles in this publication, please contact the Commercial Reprints Department, Elsevier Inc., 360 Park Avenue South, New York, NY 10010-1710. Tel.: 212-633-3812; Fax: 212-462-1935; E-mail: reprints@elsevier.com.

Printed and bound in the United Kingdom
Transferred to Digital Print 2011

Contributors

CONSULTING EDITOR

MARK S. MYERSON, MD
Director, Attending Orthopaedic Surgeon, The Institute for Foot and Ankle Reconstruction, Mercy Medical Center, Baltimore, Maryland

GUEST EDITOR

DAVID A. PORTER, MD, PhD
Voluntary Clinical Associate Faculty of Orthopaedics, Methodist Sports Medicine, The Orthopaedic Specialists; Faculty, Department of Orthopaedics Indiana University School of Medicine, Indianapolis, Indiana

AUTHORS

ANNUNZIATO AMENDOLA, MD
Professor, Department of Orthopaedics and Rehabilitation, University of Iowa Sports Medicine; Director, University of Iowa Sports Medicine, University of Iowa, Iowa City, Iowa

ROBERT B. ANDERSON, MD
Chief, Foot and Ankle Service, OrthoCarolina Foot and Ankle Institute; Vice Chief, Department of Orthopaedic Surgery, Carolinas Medical Center, Charlotte, North Carolina

GREGORY C. BERLET, MD
Chief, Department of Orthopaedics, Division of Foot and Ankle, Orthopaedic Foot and Ankle Center, Ohio State University, Columbus, Ohio

REBECCA A. CERRATO, MD
Attending Orthopaedic Surgeon, The Institute for Foot and Ankle Reconstruction, Mercy Medical Center, Baltimore, Maryland

MICHAEL J. COUGHLIN, MD
Clinical Professor of Orthopaedic Surgery, Oregon Health Sciences, Portland, Oregon; Idaho Foot and Ankle Fellowship, Boise, Idaho

MATTHEW DɛORIO, MD
The Orthopaedic Center, Huntsville, Alabama

MARK EASLEY, MD
Attending Physician of Orthopaedic Surgery, Duke Health Center, Durham, North Carolina

MELISSA ERICKSON, MD
Duke University Medical Center, Durham, North Carolina

CAROL FREY, MD
Co-Director, West Coast Sports Medicine Foundation Fellowship; Director, Orthopaedic Foot and Ankle Surgery; Assistant (Volunteer) Clinical Professor, Orthopaedic Surgery, University of California Los Angeles, Manhattan Beach, California

J. ADAM JELINEK, MD
Methodist Sports Medicine Center, The Orthopaedic Specialists Center, Indianapolis, Indiana

MARK A. KRAHE, DO
Fellow, Department of Orthopaedics, Ohio State University, Orthopaedic Foot and Ankle Center, Columbus, Ohio

JEFFREY A. MANN, MD
Department of Orthopaedic Surgery, Summit Medical Center, Oakland, California

ANGUS M. McBRYDE, Jr., MD
Staff Orthopaedic Surgeon, Andrews Sports Medicine and Orthopaedic Center; Director, Foot and Ankle Fellowship Program, American Sports Medicine Institute, Birmingham, Alabama

JEREMY J. McCORMICK, MD
Fellow, Foot and Ankle Surgery, OrthoCarolina Foot and Ankle Institute, Charlotte, North Carolina

MARK S. MYERSON, MD
Director, The Institute for Foot and Ankle Reconstruction, Mercy Medical Center, Baltimore, Maryland

LUDOVICO PANARELLA, MD, PhD
Associate, Department of Orthopaedics and Traumatology, Knee Surgery, Arthroscopy and Sports Medicine, University of Rome Tor Vergata, Rome, Italy

DAVID I. PEDOWITZ, MD, MS
Department of Orthopaedic Surgery, Crystal Run Healthcare, Middletown, New York

DAVID A. PORTER, MD, PhD
Voluntary Clinical Associate Faculty of Orthopaedics, Methodist Sports Medicine Center, The Orthopaedic Specialists Center; Faculty, Department of Orthopaedics, Indiana University School of Medicine, Indianapolis, Indiana

ROBERT C. SCHENCK, Jr., MD
Professor and Chairman, Department of Orthopaedic Surgery, University of New Mexico School of Medicine; Head Team Physician, University of New Mexico Lobos, Albuquerque, New Mexico

E. PEPPER TOOMEY, MD
Proliance Surgeons, Swedish Orthopaedic Institute, Seattle, Washington

FEDERICO G. USUELLI, MD
IRCCS Galeazzi, Divisione di Chirurgia del Piede e della Caviglia, Milano, Italy

Contents

The Great Toe: Failed Turf Toe, Chronic Turf Toe, and Complicated Sesamoid Injuries   **135**

Jeremy J. McCormick and Robert B. Anderson

> Turf toe injuries and sesamoid injuries are challenging because of the variety of causes that exist as sources of pain. Through a systematic approach to evaluation, injuries to the hallux metatarsophalangeal joint can be diagnosed properly. Correct diagnosis leads to accurate and efficient treatment. If conservative measures fail, operative interventions are available to relieve pain and restore function. With careful surgical technique and appropriate postoperative management, athletes can return to play and efficiently reach their pre-injury level of participation.

The Complicated Jones Fracture, Including Revision and Malalignment   **151**

Angus M. McBryde, Jr.

> Using radiographs culled over a 33-month period, the treatment, complications, revision, and rehabilitation of complicated Jones fractures and stress fractures involving the proximal diaphysis are examined. Although the non-operative approach remains viable, the exigencies and desires of the athletic and leg-based working population require sooner-rather-than-later return to play or work. Fortunately, these needs can be matched by the available and functioning orthopedic practice of intramedullary screw fixation. This practice is coupled with prevention, reliable orthopedic techniques, the orthopedist's surgical skills, and devices necessary for successful surgery. Recent attention directed toward handling complications promise better, quicker, and more reliable recovery for the patient.

Lisfranc Injuries in Sport   **169**

Matthew DeOrio, Melissa Erickson, Federico Giuseppe Usuelli, and Mark Easley

> Injuries to the Lisfranc ligament complex have traditionally been associated with high energy trauma such as motor vehicle collisions and industrial accidents. Recently, there has been a greater appreciation of mid-foot sprains that represent a spectrum of injury to the Lisfranc ligament complex. As a result, there has been an increased incidence of such injury

resulting from low-energy trauma in activities ranging from recreational activity to elite athletic activity. This article discusses issues related to anatomy, clinical presentation, mechanism of injury, and diagnosis that are necessary to provide appropriate treatment for these injuries. There should be a high index of suspicion of this injury, and prompt diagnosis is important to allow athletes to return to sport with the best possible outcome.

Despite increased awareness of stress fractures of the tarsal navicular and a heightened index of suspicion by those physicians evaluating sports related foot pain, these injuries remain difficult to diagnose. There is often a considerable delay in the diagnosis because of its subtle and often vague clinical presentation. Accompanying a thorough history and physical, the authors recommend plain radiographs of the foot and ankle, followed by a CT scan to fully characterize any fracture of the navicular and to rule out other etiologies of foot pain. If a CT scan is negative, and a high clinical suspicion persists, an MRI scan is then obtained to rule out a stress reaction. While often successful, non-operative treatment of navicular stress fractures is prolonged and often frustrating to the competitive athlete; surgical intervention for appropriately selected patients can result in full symptom resolution and a return to the desired level of athletic participation.

Ankle instability in the athlete is a common problem that is routinely treated non-operatively, with a 90% success rate. With proprioceptive training, preventive equipment (bracing/taping), and closed kinetic chain strengthening, surgery for ankle instability is uncommon. Nonetheless, some athletes present with recurrent ankle instability that, despite work-up and conservative treatment, requires surgical correction. The use of a primary ligament repair (Brostrom procedure) versus augmented (anatomic) reconstructions is discussed in detail in this article.

Chronic giving way and ankle dysfunction are common after ankle sprains. In our approach to chronic ankle pain and giving way, one must consider the differential diagnosis before treatment can be directed appropriately. One of the common diagnoses associated with ankle injury is osteochondral lesions of the talus. The advent of MRI has allowed us to make the diagnosis of occult lesions more readily. Arthroscopic and open management of these lesions continues to evolve. This article discusses osteochondral lesions of the talus, treatment options, and resurfacing techniques.

E. Pepper Toomey

Plantar fasciitis is a common problem without known etiology. It responds well to multiple conservative modalities and no particular modality has been demonstrated to be clearly superior in the treatment of this condition. Over 90% of patients will be cured by non-operative treatment but this may require 6 to 12 months of treatment and encouragement by the physician. Extracorporeal shock wave therapy is a noninvasive treatment with a success rate comparable to surgery and a low complication rate. Surgery can be done endoscopically or open with similar long-term outcomes. Patients appear to recover from endoscopic treatment 4 to 5 weeks earlier than the open group. If there is a suggestion of FBLPN entrapment, then patients should have an open release.

Mark A. Krahe and Gregory C. Berlet

Achilles tendon pathology is one of the more common conditions encountered by the foot and ankle surgeon. While it most frequently affects the athletic population, it can also lead to significant morbidity in the older and sedentary patient. The etiology of Achilles tendon dysfunction is multifactorial and has been found to be associated with overuse injury, training error, malalignment of the lower extremity, inflammatory disorders, and intrinsic disease or degeneration. Achilles tendon disorders have been classified temporally as acute and chronic, with the later subdivided into insertional and non-insertional (intrinsic) involvement. Histopathology has contributed a great deal to the understanding of disease process. Classification systems have been developed in an attempt to determine methods of treatment and prognosis. This article reviews the clinical spectrum of disease and presents contemporary treatment options.

J. Adam Jelinek and David A. Porter

Athletes with unstable ankle injuries treated with rigid and anatomic internal fixation with concomitant repair of indicated ligaments followed by an accelerated rehabilitation program consisting of early weight bearing and near-immediate range of motion (ROM) can obtain excellent outcomes. Early ROM and weight bearing, if indicated depending on the specific injury pattern, can be effective with low morbidity. Return to sports can be expected as early as 4 weeks after rigid fixation of an isolated fibula fracture and up to 8 to 10 weeks after stabilization of a bimalleolar equivalent fracture with deltoid repair. Syndesmosis fixation can take up to 4 to 6 months before successful return to sport.

THE CLINICS ARE NOW AVAILABLE ONLINE!

Access your subscription at:
www.theclinics.com

Foreword

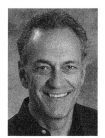

Mark S. Myerson, MD
Consulting Editor

What are your goals for treatment of the athlete? Who is an athlete? Today, more and more patients consider themselves athletically active, and indeed some of the articles in this issue address these specific individuals who suffer from activity- and stress-related injuries. Many other patients, however, have variants of these problems (ie, tendinosis, bone impingement, arthritis) which are not in any way caused, but aggravated and made more symptomatic by the sporting activity.

What changes have you, the reader, noted over the past decade in your orthopedic practice? Have these changes been related to or driven by changes in technology, new surgical techniques, or changes in the *demographics* of a particular pathology such as stress fractures? All of these changes probably apply to the management of athletic injury of the foot and ankle, but I have been impressed mostly by technological advances which have facilitated the treatment of these conditions. Take as an example the management of insertional Achilles tendinopathy. The basic principles of treatment have not changed much: aggressively remove all degenerated necrotic tissue, remove all the impinging bone and then re-attach the tendon to the calcaneus with or without the addition of a tendon transfer (the flexor hallucis longus). However, it has been the subtle change to treatment made available by the use of specific suture anchors which have facilitated the re-attachment of the tendon to the bone, and a far more rapid recovery for the patient. This applies as well to the management of stress fractures, for example, of the fifth metatarsal and the type of fixation used. We have recognized that early percutaneous fixation of a stress fracture of the fifth metatatarsal speeds up the patient's recovery and return to sports, but it has been the technologic changes with respect to the type of screw fixation and how this is supplemented with bone stimulation which has facilitated recovery.

The contributors to this issue all have extensive experience with the treatment of athletic foot and ankle injury ranging from the professional to the high school athlete. To some extent the principles of treating a problem, for example a stress fracture, are the same regardless of the type of athlete. The pressures on everyone, including the surgeon, the athlete, and the members of the team are all very different, emphasizing

Foot Ankle Clin N Am 14 (2009) xi–xii
doi:10.1016/j.fcl.2009.03.002
1083-7515/09/$ – see front matter © 2009 Elsevier Inc. All rights reserved.

foot.theclinics.com

a need to understand the dynamics of maximizing the return of an athlete to his or her sport. This must be done however without compromising the final outcome. Whether the pressure is applied by an anxious parent or the player, the surgeon must not jeopardize the treatment nor the rehabilitation in order to expedite recovery.

Mark S. Myerson, MD
Director, Institute for Foot and Ankle Reconstruction
Mercy Medical Center
301 St. Paul Place
Baltimore, MD 21202, USA

E-mail address:
Mark4feet@aol.com (M.S. Myerson)

Preface

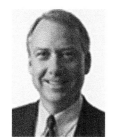

David A. Porter, MD, PhD
Guest Editor

The popularity of the field of sports medicine continues to grow, and in sports medicine the specialty area of foot and ankle is particularly exciting. Foot and ankle injuries continue to be reported at an increasing rate in sports, especially in the National Football League. Great toe injuries and Lisfranc midfoot ruptures can be career-ending injuries. Achilles tendon overuse injuries as well as ruptures and peroneal tendon dislocations and tears continue to plague the athletes and clinicians alike. Plantar fasciitis is almost epidemic in the National Basketball Association, and ankle fractures in the athlete are common but poorly described in the literature. Equally enigmatic are the navicular stress fracture and the Jones fracture of the fifth metatarsal. This issue has an excellent chapter on osteochondral lesions of the talus that provides a clear picture of diagnosing and treating this sometime difficult entity. We hope this issue of the *Foot and Ankle Clinics of North America* will help the reader and clinicians in diagnosing, treating, and rehabilitating the athlete who have foot and ankle injuries. We have asked our distinguished specialists trained in foot and ankle injuries to discuss these areas in the more complicated cases. For instance, a great deal has been written about ankle sprains in the athletes, but questions remain about the effective treatment of the large-framed (> 250 pounds) athlete who has chronic lateral instability, inherent ligamentous laxity, a varus hindfoot, or a failed prior lateral ligamentous reconstruction. Another thorny question is the best treatment for syndesmosis injury in the athlete, both acute and chronic. Discussions of these issues, and more, are in this issue highlighting complicated foot and ankle problems in the athlete. Enjoy and be up to date!

David A. Porter, MD, PhD
Methodist Sports Medicine
6350 East 10th Street
Fishers, IN 46038, USA

E-mail address:
davidaporter@sbcglobal.net (D.A. Porter)

Foot Ankle Clin N Am 14 (2009) xiii
doi:10.1016/j.fcl.2009.04.002
1083-7515/09/$ – see front matter © 2009 Elsevier Inc. All rights reserved.

The Great Toe: Failed Turf Toe, Chronic Turf Toe, and Complicated Sesamoid Injuries

Jeremy J. McCormick, MD[a], Robert B. Anderson, MD[a,b],*

KEYWORDS

• Turf toe • Sesamoids • Great toe • Hallux • Injury
• Hallux metatarsophalangeal joint

Great toe injuries often are underappreciated and can lead to significant functional disability. Among university athletes, Clanton and Ford[1] found that foot injuries were the third leading cause of missed time and that a large portion of these injuries involved the hallux metatarsophalangeal (MTP) joint. Turf toe and sesamoid injury are two such entities that require accurate diagnosis and management. If unrecognized or mistreated, they can lead to chronic problems such as loss of push-off strength, persistent pain, progressive deformity, and, eventually, joint degeneration. This article focuses on the complex great toe, addressing issues such as failed turf toe treatment, chronic turf toe injuries, and complicated sesamoid injuries such as non-union and avascular necrosis (AVN).

ANATOMY

The hallux MTP joint does not have inherent stability because the proximal phalanx has a shallow cavity in which the metatarsal head articulates. Most of the stability comes from the capsular ligamentous sesamoid complex (**Fig. 1**). Fan-shaped medial and lateral collateral ligaments course between the proximal phalanx and the metatarsal. Each is composed of an MTP ligament and a metatarso-sesamoid ligament. The collateral ligaments are important for stability of the MTP joint in cutting activities. The plantar plate is a separate fibrous structure that courses from a firm attachment on the proximal phalanx to a weaker attachment, through the joint

[a] OrthoCarolina Foot and Ankle Institute, 1001 Blythe Boulevard, Suite 200, Charlotte, NC 28203, USA
[b] Foot and Ankle Service, Department of Orthopaedic Surgery, Carolinas Medical Center, PO Box 32861, Charlotte, NC 28232, USA
* Corresponding author. OrthoCarolina Foot and Ankle Institute, 1001 Blythe Boulevard, Suite 200, Charlotte, NC 28203, USA.
E-mail address: robert.anderson@orthocarolina.com (R.B. Anderson).

Foot Ankle Clin N Am 14 (2009) 135–150
doi:10.1016/j.fcl.2009.01.001
1083-7515/09/$ – see front matter © 2009 Elsevier Inc. All rights reserved.

foot.theclinics.com

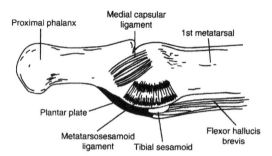

Fig. 1. Medial aspect of the first metatarsophalangeal joint. *From* Bowman MW. Athletic injuries of the great to metatarsophalangeal joint. In: Adelaar RS, editor. Disorders of the Great toe. Rosemont (IL): American Academy of Orthopaedic Surgeons; 1997. p. 3. (Copyright © 1996, Michael W. Bowman, MD; with permission.)

capsule, to the metatarsal head. In fact, the capsular ligamentous complex of the MTP joint is a confluence of structures including the collateral ligaments and plantar plate, as well as the abductor hallucis, adductor hallucis, and flexor hallucis brevis (FHB).

The FHB originates from the plantar aspect of the cuboid and lateral cuneiform as well as from the posterior tibialis insertion over the medial and middle cuneiforms. Moving distally, the FHB divides into medial and lateral tendons that envelop the medial (tibial) and lateral (fibular) sesamoid, respectively. At the level of the sesamoids, the abductor hallucis tendon conjoins with the medial head of the FHB tendon, and the adductor hallucis tendon conjoins with the lateral head of the FHB tendon. The FHB tendons then insert at the base of the proximal phalanx with the thick volar (plantar) plate as part of the capsular ligamentous complex.

The sesamoid bones typically ossify between the ages of 9 and 11 years, often with multiple sites of ossification. The medial sesamoid is larger and longer than the lateral sesamoid and tends to rest more distally. In addition to being larger, the medial sesamoid often is situated more directly under the metatarsal head, thus sustaining greater weight bearing forces. The sesamoids form an articulating joint with the metatarsal head and are connected by the intersesamoid ligament. Their function is to dissipate force at the MTP joint and to provide a mechanical advantage for the FHB by elevating the metatarsal head. Last, the sesamoids help protect the flexor hallucis longus (FHL) and maintain its course along the plantar aspect of the great toe.

The capsular ligamentous sesamoid complex of the hallux MTP must withstand 40% to 60% of body weight during normal gait.[2] During athletic activity, this force increases to two to three times body weight, and, with a running jump, the forces at the MTP joint complex can reach eight times body weight.[3] These data show that the capsular ligamentous sesamoid complex is critical to the function of an athlete and indicate the importance of careful consideration in the care of hallux MTP joint injuries.

TURF TOE INJURIES

A turf toe injury is a sprain or tear of the capsular ligamentous structure of the first MTP joint. It originally was described by Bowers and Martin[4] in 1976, who found an average of 5.4 turf toe injuries per football season in football players at the University of West Virginia. Similar numbers were found by Coker and colleagues[5] at the University of Arkansas and by Clanton and colleagues[6] at Rice University, who found 6.0 and 4.5 turf toe injuries per football season, respectively. In 1990, Rodeo and colleagues[7] published a survey of 80 active players in the National Football League. They found that

45% of the players had experienced a turf toe injury, and 83% of those injuries occurred on artificial turf. Although the injury classically occurs in football players participating on artificial surfaces, turf toe injuries can occur in any field sport and on any surface. There has been an apparent increase in the occurrence of turf toe injuries, possibly because of the use of more flexible, lighter shoes or changes in surface–cleat interaction.

The typical mechanism of most turf toe injuries is delivery of an axial load to a foot that is in fixed equinus. The load drives the hallux MTP joint into hyperextension, leading to attenuation or disruption of the plantar joint complex (**Fig. 2**). A spectrum of injuries can occur, ranging from strain or sprain of plantar structures to frank dorsal dislocation of the toe. With unrestricted dorsiflexion, further injury can occur to the joint surface or subchondral bone as the proximal phalanx impacts on the dorsal aspect of the metatarsal head.

Variations of the typical turf toe injury are based on the position of the hallux and the force of injury. The most common variant, described by Watson and colleagues,[8] involves a valgus-directed force which results in greater injury to the medial/plantar-medial ligamentous structures and tibial sesamoid complex. Douglas and colleagues[9] reported on a case of this type in which a soccer player was slide-tackled from the side. After conservative treatment for his hallux MTP injury was unsuccessful, the player obtained an MRI that showed a medial collateral ligament injury of the great toe requiring repair. In some cases, injuries to the medial structures allow lateral contracture, leading to a traumatic hallux valgus and bunion deformity as a result of unbalanced force from the adductor hallucis tendon. Hallux varus deformity also has been reported from a traumatic blow to the hallux MTP joint causing injury to the plantar lateral structures of the capsular ligamentous complex.

Evaluation

Turf toe represents a broad spectrum of injury with degrees of soft tissue injury ranging from ligament strain to frank dislocation of the MTP joint. The category of turf toe has been grouped into hyperextension, hyperflexion, and dislocation injuries, which usually can be distinguished by the history and physical examination (**Table 1**). Additionally, to guide treatment and return to play, a clinical classification has been devised (**Table 2**). Because of the variability in degree and type of injury, it is important to evaluate any turf toe carefully. To determine the type or extent of injury, it is helpful to understand the mechanism and timing surrounding the occurrence. Additionally, it is important to evaluate a turf toe injury acutely, because the acute examination can be more helpful in localizing injured structures.

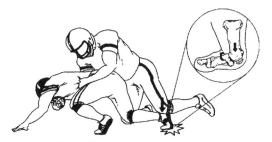

Fig. 2. Foot in fixed equinus with axially directed load leading to turf toe injury. *From* Bowman MW. Athletic injuries of the great to metatarsophalangeal joint. In: Adelaar RS, editor. Disorders of the Great toe. Rosemont (IL): American Academy of Orthopaedic Surgeons; 1997. p. 8. (Copyright © 1996, Michael W. Bowman, MD; with permission.)

Table 1
Classification of turf toe injury

Type of Injury	Grade	Description
Hyperextension (turf toe)	I	Stretching of plantar capsular ligamentous complex
		Localized tenderness, minimal swelling, minimal ecchymosis
	II	Partial tear of plantar capsular ligamentous complex
		Diffuse tenderness, moderate swelling, ecchymosis
		Restricted movement with pain
	III	Frank tear of plantar capsular ligamentous complex
		Severe tenderness, marked swelling and ecchymosis
		Limited movement with pain, plus vertical Lachman's test
		Possible associated injuries:
		Medial/lateral injury
		Sesamoid fracture/bipartite diastasis
		Articular cartilage/subchondral bone bruise
Hyperflexion (sand toe)	—	Hyperflexion injury to hallux MTP or IP joint
		May involve injury to lesser MTP joints as well
Dislocation	I	Dislocation of the hallux with the sesamoids
		No disruption of the intersesamoid ligament
		Frequently irreducible
	IIA	Associated disruption of the intersesamoid ligament
		Usually reducible
	IIB	Associated transverse fracture of one or both sesamoids
		Usually reducible
	IIC	Complete disruption of intersesamoid ligament with fracture of one of the sesamoids
		Usually reducible

From Anderson RB, Shawen SB. Great toe disorders. In: Porter DA, Schon LC, editors. Baxter's the foot and ankle in sport. 2nd edition. Philadelphia: Elsevier Health Sciences; 2007. p. 423; with permission. (*Adapted from* Adelaar RS, editor. Disorders of the great toe. Rosemont (IL): American Academy of Orthopaedic Surgeons; 1997; with permission.)

The assessment should begin with observation of the hallux MTP joint for ecchymosis or swelling. This observation should be followed by a careful, systematic palpation of the capsular ligamentous structures, namely the collateral ligaments, dorsal capsule, and plantar sesamoid complex. The MTP joint then should be trialed through a series of range of motion maneuvers to determine instability. Varus and valgus stress can be placed on the joint to determine the integrity of the collateral ligaments. Decreased resistance to dorsiflexion suggests a plantar plate injury. A dorso-plantar drawer test, similar to the Lachman test at the knee, is another maneuver that contributes important information about the integrity of the joint capsule. Next, active flexion and extension of the MTP joint should be evaluated to determine the integrity of the flexor and extensor tendons. Grading the strength of hallux MTP active flexion can be helpful in determining the extent of injury, because normal strength suggests a less severe structural injury. One should remember, however, that the assessment of an acutely injured athlete may be difficult because of the discomfort or pain of the trauma.

Once the physical examination is completed, radiographic evaluation is mandatory for hyperextension injuries. One should obtain weight bearing anteroposterior and lateral views of the foot as well as a sesamoid axial view. Most often, the radiographs

Grade	Objective Findings	Activity Level	Treatment
	Table 2		
	Clinical classification system for turf toe injury		
1	Localized planter or medial tenderness Minimal swelling No ecchymosis	Continued athletic participation	Symptomatic
2	More diffuse and intense tenderness Mild to moderate swelling Mild to moderate ecchymosis	Loss of playing time for 3–14 days	Walking boot and crutches as needed
3	Severe and diffuse tenderness Marked swelling Moderate to severe ecchymosis Painful and limited range of motion	Loss of playing time for at least 4–6 weeks	Long-term immobilization in boot or cast versus surgical repair

From Anderson RB, Shawen SB. Great toe disorders. In: Porter DA, Schon LC, editors. Baxter's the foot and ankle in sport. 2nd edition. Philadelphia: Elsevier Health Sciences; 2007. p. 424; with permission. (*Adapted from* Adelaar RS, editor. Disorders of the great toe. Rosemont (IL): American Academy of Orthopaedic Surgeons; 1997; with permission.)

are negative; however, one may find a small avulsion fracture from the plantar aspect of the proximal phalanx or the distal aspect of a sesamoid. This finding would suggest a capsular avulsion. Comparison with radiographs of the contralateral, uninjured foot is highly recommended, because Prieskorn and colleagues[10] reported that patients who had complete rupture of the plantar plate would have proximal migration of the sesamoids. Absolute evaluation measurements are 10.4 mm from the distal tip of the tibial sesamoid to the joint and 13.3 mm from the distal tip of the fibular sesamoid to the joint. Measurements greater than these distances have a 99.7% chance of plantar plate rupture.[8]

If there is clinical suspicion for a plantar plate injury, a forced dorsiflexion lateral radiograph, described by Rodeo and colleagues,[7] can be obtained. With passive hyperextension of the hallux MTP joint, the sesamoids should migrate distally. The forced dorsiflexion lateral radiograph helps assess this movement and delineates diastasis of a fractured or bipartite sesamoid, joint subluxation, or proximal sesamoid migration in the case of a more serious plantar plate injury. Whenever possible, fluoroscopic imaging is used to produce a real-time view of the MTP joint and sesamoid complex. The injured toe is examined for integrity of the plantar plate through dynamic motion and is compared with the contralateral side. Much as with the forced dorsiflexion lateral view, lack of distal sesamoid excursion with toe extension suggests the plantar soft tissue disruption. Live fluoroscopy is both diagnostic and educational to the patient in demonstrating the turf toe injury. In the authors' practice, the use of fluoroscopy has become a standard part of the diagnostic algorithm.

In addition to plain radiographs and fluoroscopy, arthrography was used historically as an adjunctive study. Although arthrography, particularly in the acute injury, still may be the best method of identifying the presence or extent of a capsular disruption, MRI has replaced it in most circumstances. MRI can be used to identify soft tissue injury as well as osseous or articular damage. T2-weighted images obtained in coronal, axial, and sagittal planes provide an optimum level of anatomic detail and identify subtle injury.[11] An MRI should be obtained in all grade 2 or 3 injuries, because it provides critical information to help formulate a treatment plan and prognosis. **Fig. 3** shows a sagittal spectral presaturation inversion recovery (SPIR) image of the hallux MTP joint with clear disruption of the plantar capsular ligamentous structures just distal to the sesamoid bone.

Treatment

Once the turf toe is recognized, treatment in the early stages is similar for all grades of injury. The basic principles of rest, ice, compression, and elevation (RICE) can be applied to help reduce initial swelling.[1] Additionally, an anti-inflammatory medication can be used to help relieve symptoms. Taping is not advised in the acute setting because it may compromise circulation. In addition to RICE, athletes may benefit from the use of a walking boot or a short leg cast with a toe spica extension in slight plantarflexion. The spica extension protects the hallux from extension at the MTP joint while theoretically bringing the plantar rupture into close apposition. With this protection in place, the patient may bear weight as tolerated. If symptoms permit, gentle range of motion exercises can begin at 3 to 5 days from the injury. As early treatment continues, it is important to complete the diagnostic process and grade the injury to help direct continued treatment and prognosis for return to play. Cortisone or anesthetic injections are not advised.

A grade 1 injury, or plantar structure attenuation, allows athletes to return to competition with little or no loss of playing time. The toe may benefit from taping in slight plantarflexion to provide compression and limit movement. In addition, the athlete should modify his or her shoewear to a stiff-soled shoe that includes a turf toe plate to limit hallux MTP extension. Another option is a custom orthotic with a Morton's extension. Many runners or football "skill position" athletes resist the shoewear modifications because of a perceived loss of mobility.

A grade 2 injury, or partial plantar capsular ligamentous rupture, generally results in a loss of playing time of at least 2 weeks. The same treatment regimen used for grade 1 injuries should be applied to grade 2 injuries. Return to play is dictated by the athlete's symptoms and ability to reach near preinjury level of performance.

A grade 3 injury, or complete plantar capsular ligamentous rupture, may require up to 8 weeks of recovery. With these injuries, a longer period of immobilization is appropriate before return to play. Again, return is dictated by symptoms, but ideally, the hallux MTP joint will have 50° to 60° of painless passive dorsiflexion. Additionally, the requirements of an athlete's sport or position play a role in determining ability to return to activity. For example, a football cornerback probably would return later than a lineman with a similar injury because of the increased demands for push-off and cutting required by the cornerback position. It should be made clear to the athlete,

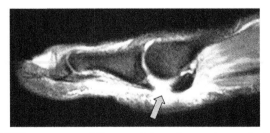

Fig. 3. T2 sagittal SPIR sequence of the great toe. Arrow demonstrates rupture of the capsular ligamentous complex just distal to the medial sesamoid bone.

however, that a recovery period of up to 6 months can be expected before symptoms resolve completely and shoewear modifications and taping are not necessary.

Turf toe injuries and their recovery can be challenging and frustrating. Fortunately, operative treatment seldom is necessary. The decision to treat a patient surgically is a difficult one. Indications for surgery are listed in **Box 1**.

Classically, acute repair or reconstruction of the plantar capsular ligamentous complex of the hallux MTP has been performed through a medial incision or a J incision, in which the medial incision is extended horizontally across the hallux MTP flexion crease. With this approach, care must be taken to identify and protect the plantarmedial digital nerve as it courses near the tibial sesamoid. The soft tissues are freed carefully to identify the defect in the plantar plate that typically is distal to the sesamoids. Plantarflexion of the joint can assist in visualization of the defect. Once identified, the gap in the ruptured capsular ligamentous complex is primarily repaired with nonabsorbable sutures. Usually, one finds adequate tissue on the base of the proximal phalanx for reattachment. If this tissue is inadequate, suture anchors or drill holes can be used to assure firm fixation of the soft tissues to the proximal phalanx. In making the repair, one must be sure to avoid suturing the FHL tendon, because it is intimately involved with the plantar complex of the MTP joint.

Recently, the authors have been using a two-incision technique for improved access to the lateral aspect of the plantar plate (**Fig. 4**). With this method, the medial approach and exposure is completed exactly as in the classic approach, but without the "J" extension of the incision across the flexion crease. Again, care is taken to protect the plantarmedial digital nerve (**Fig. 5**). Once the plantar defect is identified and exposed, the second incision is made just lateral to the fibular sesamoid. This incision is slightly curved to follow the soft tissue contour of the fat pad of the hallux MTP and avoid symptomatic scar formation. The soft tissue is dissected with care taken to identify and protect the common plantar digital nerve and its proper plantar branch to the lateral aspect of the great toe. Much as on the medial side, the defect in the capsular ligamentous complex can be identified, typically just distal to the fibular sesamoid. Once the soft tissues are freed, one has excellent access to the hallux MTP joint from medial and lateral sides and can begin the plantar plate repair with nonabsorbable sutures.

Beginning through the lateral incision, sutures should be placed from deep to superficial. That is, a suture should be placed to repair the joint capsule starting from a point

---

Box 1
Indications for surgical repair of turf toe injury

1. Large capsular avulsion with unstable joint
2. Diastasis of bipartite sesamoid
3. Diastasis of sesamoid fracture
4. Retraction of sesamoid(s)
5. Traumatic hallux valgus deformity
6. Vertical instability (positive Lachman's test)
7. Loose body
8. Chondral injury
9. Failed conservative treatment

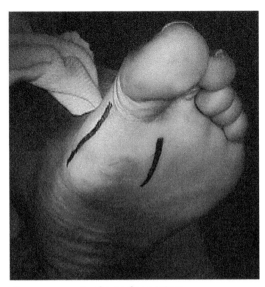

Fig. 4. Two incisions for open repair of a turf toe injury.

deep in the lateral incision, at the midline of the MTP joint, near the FHL tendon. Suturing should continue in interrupted fashion toward the most lateral extent of the MTP joint. Generally three or four sutures are used. Sutures should be passed through the full thickness of soft tissue that is available. Care should be taken to pass a suture to a point directly opposite its start to avoid the pronation or supination of the toe that might occur with medial or lateral advancement of a suture pass. Each suture should be tagged after placement, because tying should occur after all sutures, both medial and lateral, have been placed. After the sutures are placed through the lateral wound, a similar method of suture repair is performed through the medial wound for the medial aspect of the joint capsule. Once all of the sutures are in place (**Fig. 6**A, B), they are tied in the order they were inserted (**Fig. 6**C). Care should be taken to place the hallux MTP joint in approximately 15° of plantarflexion as the sutures are tied. After repair,

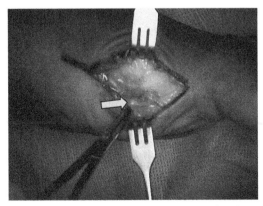

Fig. 5. Medial exposure with arrow identifying the plantarmedial digital nerve.

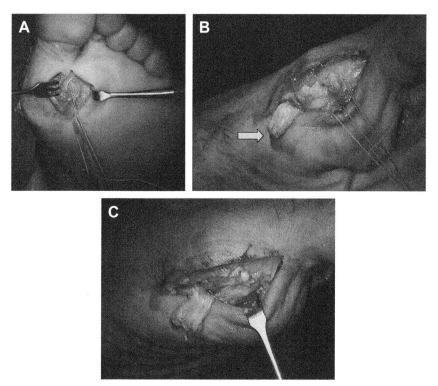

Fig. 6. (*A*) Lateral exposure with sutures in place. (*B*) Medial exposure with sutures in place. Arrow points to the abductor hallucis tendon, which was avulsed in this patient's injury. (*C*) Medial view with sutures tied (three knots are visible).

intraoperative fluoroscopy can be used to verify an improved, advanced position of the sesamoids as well as fluid excursion of the sesamoids with hallux MTP dorsiflexion.

If the turf toe injury is a medial-based soft tissue injury, surgical management can consist of a procedure similar to that of a modified McBride bunionectomy. This procedure involves excising the medial eminence of the metatarsal head and repairing the overlying soft tissue rupture through a medial incision. In addition, an incision in the dorsal first web space is used to release the adductor hallucis tendon in an effort to minimize potential deforming forces on the MTP joint.

When there is a sesamoid fracture or diastasis of a bipartite sesamoid, the authors recommend preserving one pole of the sesamoid, if possible. Ideally, there is a smaller distal pole fragment that is amenable to excision. Once the bone is excised, the remaining soft tissues are repaired using drill holes through the remaining proximal sesamoid as an adjunct. If complete sesamoidectomy is necessary, a large soft tissue defect may remain within the plantar complex, subsequently compromising flexor power or resulting in a fixed deformity. In this situation, the abductor hallucis tendon can be detached from its distal insertion, mobilized, and transferred plantarly into the defect. This transfer provides collagen for structural stability, thereby improving plantar restraint to dorsiflexion forces and augmenting the flexion power of the hallux MTP joint.

Late reconstruction of a turf toe injury may be necessary in an athlete who is inadequately diagnosed or treated or in the athlete who continues to perform despite injury. As a result of unrestrained dorsiflexion, secondary hallux MTP disorders can occur such as longitudinal tears of the FHL tendon or hallux rigidus with joint degeneration from repetitive joint impaction. Other sequelae include a progressive hallux valgus or varus deformity or cock-up toe with a hallux interphalangeal (IP) joint flexion contracture. In these situations, surgical reconstruction is difficult because of retraction and scarring of the soft tissues. Advancement of the capsule and sesamoids may require fasciotomies or fractional lengthening of the proximal FHB and/or abductor hallucis muscle-tendon unit. For hallux rigidus–type symptoms, one should consider a joint debridement with cheilectomy in addition to any necessary soft tissue repair or reconstruction.

As mentioned earlier, late sequelae of turf toe injuries may include the development of a claw-toe or cock-up toe deformity with IP joint flexion contracture. If the IP and MTP joints remain passively correctable, a flexor-to-extensor transfer can be performed to reposition the toe. This transfer can be accomplished with a Girdlestone-Taylor type procedure, splitting the flexor tendon and re-approximating it into the dorsal extensor complex or directly transferring the flexor tendon through a drill hole in the proximal phalanx and securing it with a biotenodesis screw. If the IP joint has developed a fixed contracture, then, in addition to the flexor to extensor tendon transfer, the IP joint is arthrodesed.

Postoperative management of surgical reconstruction is challenging because finding a balance between soft tissue protection and early range of motion is difficult. All patients need careful monitoring and care from athletic trainers and physical therapists. Immediately after surgery, the toe should remain immobilized in 5° to 10° of plantarflexion. A toe spica splint is useful in this regard. With careful supervision to avoid excessive dorsiflexion, gentle passive range of motion maneuvers can begin at 5 to 7 days to decrease the development of arthrofibrosis at the sesamoid–metatarsal articulation. The patient should remain non–weight bearing with a removable splint or protective boot and, at night, should wear a removable bunion splint with plantar restraint. The patient may begin protective weight bearing in a boot at 4 weeks. At this point active motion can be initiated with progression over time. The patient can discontinue use of the boot 2 months after surgery and begin to use shoes modified with a plantar plate or insert to prevent hallux MTP hyperextension. The athlete is allowed to continue increasing activities as tolerated with protective taping and shoewear and can return to contact activity at 3 to 4 months. Despite a return to full activity, it should be clear to the patient that full recovery will take at least 6 months and often takes as long as 12 months.

Various authors have reported on their experience with turf toe injuries. Anderson[12] reported on 19 high level athletes that underwent evaluation for disabling turf toe injuries, nine of which were operatively repaired. All but two patients returned to full athletic activity with documented restoration of plantar stability. There were no operative complications. Coker and colleagues[5] reported on nine athletes who had a hyperextension injury to the first MTP joint, finding that the most common long-term complaints were joint stiffness and pain with athletic activity. Clanton and colleagues[6] had a larger group of 20 patients at a 5-year follow-up from a turf toe injury. Fifty percent of these athletes reported the persistence of symptoms of pain and stiffness. These reports indicate that prompt and accurate diagnosis and treatment, with surgical intervention where indicated, are important to give an athlete the best chance of a successful outcome while minimizing long-term sequelae.

SESAMOID INJURIES

Sesamoid pain has numerous causes. The most general term, "sesamoiditis," perhaps best describes a symptom rather than a diagnosis. It is defined as pain in the sesamoid region with negative radiographs and an equivocal MRI. Sesamoiditis should be considered a diagnosis of exclusion, when soft tissue problems such as bursitis and flexor tendinitis are considered first. There often is an associated history of overuse or minor trauma.[13,14]

Fracture of the sesamoid is another cause of sesamoid pain. It may be the result of an acute injury, as in a hyperextension injury or direct blow. Also, a fracture may result from stress injury, as happens in runners or aerobics instructors who have repetitive impact through the forefoot. The medial (tibial) sesamoid is involved more frequently, because it is larger and bears more weight than its lateral counterpart. The fracture line typically appears transversely across the sesamoid, at the level of the mid-waist. Sesamoid fractures can also be associated with MTP dislocation (Jahss type II).[15]

Degenerative causes for sesamoid pain include chondromalacia, impingement, or osteophyte formation. The mechanism and development of these pathologies is akin to those at the patellofemoral joint, with repetitive injury or chondral damage as an inciting event. The degeneration of the sesamoid articulation at the hallux MTP joint can occur as an isolated entity or in association with an inflammatory disorder such as gout.

Osteochondrosis is yet another reason for sesamoid pain. The exact cause often is unknown, but considerations include sequelae from a crush injury, stress fracture, or AVN of the sesamoid. AVN most frequently affects the lateral (fibular) sesamoid bone. With osteochondrosis, there often is painful fragmentation of the sesamoid and cyst formation followed by flattening of the bone. Symptoms may be present for 6 to 12 months before any changes can be visualized on radiographs.

Plantar prominence of the sesamoids can occur, typically in long-distance runners. The most frequent cause of pain in these patients is bursitis or intractable plantar keratosis (IPK), or both. Less commonly, osteomyelitis of the sesamoid can result from direct extension of an ulcer or puncture wound.[16] Tumors of the sesamoid bones are very rare, and, if present, appear more frequently in the lateral sesamoid.[15]

Evaluation

As with all athletic injuries, evaluation of sesamoid pain should begin with a complete history. Typically, the patient reports pain localized to the plantar aspect of the hallux MTP joint, particularly with weight bearing. The discomfort worsens with athletic activity or stair climbing and may not have a precipitating event. The clinical examination should follow and, with this, one can identify a specific location of pain and tenderness. Plantarmedial signs suggest the source of pain is the tibial sesamoid, whereas tenderness directly plantar to the MTP joint points more toward the fibular sesamoid. Along with tenderness to palpation, the presence of swelling, warmth, or erythema should be noted. Joint motion and stability also should be assessed; decreased motion may be caused by pain or an associated hallux rigidus. If vertical instability is present at the MTP joint, one should consider turf toe as the cause of pain. If compression of the sesamoids produces pain and grinding with motion, it suggests arthritis at the metatarso-sesamoid articulation. Presence of an IPK or sesamoid bursitis should be noted and may be the result of a plantar-flexed first ray, described by Manoli[17] as part of a subtle cavus foot posture.

After the history and examination, obtaining radiographs is mandatory in any thorough evaluation. Standing anteroposterior and lateral views should be obtained as well as axial or tangential views for improved assessment of the sesamoids and their articulation with the metatarsal head. One can see focal arthrosis, bony prominences, or plantar osteophytes more clearly with the special sesamoid views. An oblique view is more helpful in evaluating for fracture, particularly of the tibial sesamoid. Placing a marker (a metallic BB) on the skin overlying the point of maximal tenderness will help differentiate which sesamoid may be involved with pathology.

In examining radiographs for possible sesamoid fracture, one should keep in mind that as many as 33% of the population has a congenital partition of the sesamoid (bipartite). A fracture has sharp, irregular borders on both sides of the separation. A bipartite sesamoid, on the other hand, has smooth cortical edges with a relatively larger total size than a single sesamoid. Contralateral views also might be helpful, because Zinman and colleagues[18] cited up to a 90% incidence of bilateral occurrence or bipartite sesamoids.

Unfortunately, even with a thorough examination and radiographic review, the cause of sesamoid pain remains difficult to diagnose. MRI may be used because it is helpful in differentiating between bone and soft tissue abnormality. The MRI can assess sesamoid viability, joint degeneration, and tendon continuity. An additional study that may be helpful is a bone scan. Although it may have a high rate of false-positive findings, a three-phase bone scan with pinhole images is helpful in distinguishing between the medial and the lateral sesamoid as the source of pain. Last, a CT scan is optimal for defining the bony structure of the sesamoids in their articulation. The CT helps determine the degree of metatarso-sesamoid arthrosis and also helps in evaluating fracture healing.

Treatment

As with treatment of many orthopedic injuries, nonoperative management for sesamoid injuries begins with RICE. Athletes often need to modify their activity or training regimens accordingly. Analgesics or anti-inflammatory medication can be used adjunctively for additional relief. If an injury is more severe, a patient should wear a protective boot or cast but can remain weight bearing as tolerated. The cast might include a toe spica extension holding the MTP joint in slight plantarflexion to relieve stress across the sesamoids. In milder injuries, taping can be used to provide compression and limit movement. As the pain subsides and the patient returns to more normal activity, it will be helpful for the patient to modify shoewear and use orthotic devices. Off-the-shelf options include a turf toe plate that can span the full length of the foot or just the forefoot. A custom-made version of this device is a Morton's extension that limits MTP dorsiflexion of the great toe. Other inserts such as a metatarsal pad or arch support may be used just proximal to the symptomatic sesamoid to help unload some of the weight bearing forces. Patients should be counseled that shoes with low heel heights will help avoid increased pressure across the sesamoids. Last, the shoe itself might be stiffened with a plate construction built into the sole as a permanent modification. Although the authors do not advise an intra-articular cortisone or anesthetic injection for return to athletics, one might consider an anesthetic alone for pain in a single nerve distribution.

There are many surgical options for treatment of sesamoid pain when conservative management has been exhausted and failed. The choice of procedure should be directed to the patient's pathology. For instance, if an IPK develops over an area of bone prominence or plantar exostosis of a sesamoid, failure to improve with an accommodative orthosis is an indication for surgical intervention. This situation is most common with the medial sesamoid. Shaving the plantar aspect of the sesamoid, including the offending bone spur, is the procedure of choice and is performed through a plantarmedial approach. Once the sesamoid is located, the overlying periosteum should be divided and reflected for optimal exposure while maintaining the continuity of the FHB expanse. The plantar 50% of the sesamoid is resected with a microsagittal saw, and the overlying soft tissues are repaired. Care is taken to avoid injury to the FHL or violation of the joint. The patient is allowed to bear weight immediately in a hard-sole shoe. Over the next 6 to 8 weeks, as swelling and pain subside, the patient gradually can resume normal shoewear and activities.

Sesamoid fractures are another source of pain that may require surgical intervention. There have been reports of internal fixation to repair sesamoid fractures,[19] although in limited series. Stress fractures typically occur with repetitive use, such as in a long-distance runner. As a result of subtle radiographic findings, these injuries are often diagnosed well after the initial insult and may have an established non-union. In this scenario, conservative measures consist of accommodative inserts to relieve sesamoid pressure and to limit dorsiflexion. Failure to improve with this modality would lead one to consider surgical intervention. In an effort to avoid excision, successful bone grafting of non-unions has been reported.[20]

Bone grafting a sesamoid non-union can be technically challenging. It is indicated for a waist fracture that has minimal diastasis, typically less than 2 mm. It is important that the articular surface of the sesamoid is intact and free of injury and that the fracture fragments do not demonstrate gross motion between one another. Typically, the medial sesamoid sustains the stress fracture, and the surgical approach is plantarmedial. The capsule is incised along the superior border of the abductor hallucis, and the cartilage of the sesamoid is examined. If there is damage or gross motion between the fragments, a sesamoidectomy is performed. If there is no cartilage damage or gross motion, an extra-articular approach to the sesamoid is performed. The non-union site is debrided of fibrous tissue until the bone surfaces are visible, with care taken not to disrupt the articular surface. Cancellous bone is harvested through the capsulotomy site, creating a small window in the medial aspect of the metatarsal head. Harvested bone graft then is packed into the non-union site, and the overlying soft tissue and periosteum are reapproximated with absorbable suture. Internal fixation is not used. The capsulotomy is repaired, and the wound is closed. Postoperatively, the patient is placed in a splint that extends beyond the toes. The patient remains non–weight bearing for 6 weeks. A short leg cast with toe spica extension is applied at 2 weeks, and at 6 weeks the patient is allowed to bear weight in a cast or boot. A shoe modified with a turf toe plate is used at 8 weeks, and by 12 weeks the patient should be able to bear weight in a shoe without restriction. A CT then is obtained to confirm union, and, if union is successful, the patient can resume running activities. Anderson and McBryde[20] reported on a series of 21 patients who had an open bone grafting of a tibial sesamoid non-union. Nineteen of these patients went on to union and regained their preinjury level of activity.

Patients who have persisting pain that is worsened with weight bearing may have radiographs that show fragmentation of the sesamoid. This osteochondrosis can be a result of etiologies such as fracture non-union and avascular necrosis. Rest, immobilization, and orthotic devices are used as nonoperative measures, but when these measures fail, a sesamoidectomy is a reasonable surgical option to assist a patient's return to recreational activities. This procedure also is used for sesamoids with degenerative joint disease, infection, or, rarely, tumor. The patient should be informed preoperatively that sesamoidectomy may come with a loss of push-off strength. Aper and colleagues[21,22] found that with medial sesamoid excision 10% of push-off strength was lost, whereas 16% was lost with lateral sesamoid excision. If both are excised simultaneously, there is a 30% loss. In the non-athlete, this decreased push-off strength is not clinically important, but the weakness could be a detriment in elite athletes, dancers, or runners.

The tibial esamoidectomy is undertaken through a medial or plantarmedial approach. Care should be taken to avoid injury to the plantarmedial digital nerve. The approach and dissection is the same as that discussed for sesamoid non-unions. It often is helpful to assess the articular surfaces through a capsulotomy to verify degenerative disease or other condition warranting sesamoid excision. The sesamoid can be resected from within the joint or extra-articularly. The extra-articular approach is preferred because it allows the surgeon to repair the FHB tendon after excision of the bone. A careful longitudinal incision with reflection of the periosteum on the plantar aspect of the sesamoid allows excellent exposure. Once the bone to be excised is visualized, a Beaver blade is useful to free the sesamoid circumferentially from its attachments. Because of the risk of residual pain, partial sesamoid excisions are reserved for the rare case in which there is a tiny proximal or distal fragment and most of the sesamoid and its articular surface are preserved. Care must be taken to avoid injury to the FHL tendon. Once the sesamoid is excised, the soft tissue is repaired with absorbable suture.

Medial sesamoidectomy may result in a significant defect in the plantar medial soft tissue complex of the hallux MTP joint. The abductor hallucis tendon is available to be transferred into this defect to aid with joint stability and flexion strength. In this procedure, the abductor tendon is released from its distal insertion and sutured into the plantar defect. A proximal fasciotomy may be required to allow for plantar rerouting of the tendon.

In the event of a concomitant hallux valgus/bunion deformity, one should consider performing a formal bunionectomy procedure at the same time as the sesamoidectomy. Doing so minimizes the risk of a progressive valgus deformity at the hallux MTP joint that may accompany an isolated medial sesamoidectomy.

In the event of a lateral sesamoidectomy, the surgeon must decide between a dorsal or plantar incision. The dorsal approach is challenging unless the patient has a large intermetatarsal angle allowing lateral subluxation of the sesamoid complex. In this approach, a longitudinal incision is made in the first webspace, and the soft tissues are dissected until there is space for a lamina spreader to be placed between the metatarsal heads. The lateral soft tissue structures of the hallux MTP joint, namely the adductor hallucis, must be released to allow access to the lateral sesamoid. Once visualized, the fibular sesamoid can be shelled from the FHB tendon. The surgeon must avoid injury to the nerve and artery that are directly plantar to the sesamoid.

The alternative is the plantar approach, which the authors prefer because it allows direct excision of the sesamoid without dissection or disruption of the lateral soft tissue structures balancing the hallux. The approach allows direct visualization and mobilization of the plantar-lateral digital nerve. In addition, the FHB tendon can be repaired directly after bone excision, thus helping maintain the soft tissue integrity at the MTP joint. The plantar incision is curvilinear, made over the fibular sesamoid but just lateral to the weight bearing pad of the hallux MTP joint. It is important to re-approximate the skin edges of the plantar incision carefully to avoid hypertrophic scar formation on the plantar aspect of the foot.

The surgeon may encounter a situation in which both the medial and lateral sesamoid are symptomatic and with pathologic changes. In this rare occurrence, the authors have found it best to stage the sesamoidectomies to avoid the potential for a cock-up deformity. The more symptomatic or obviously pathologic sesamoid is removed initially, and, if necessary, the remaining sesamoid is excised after 1 year.

Meticulous repair of the FHB tendon is mandatory in this scenario, with the addition of an abductor transfer if necessary.

The postoperative dressing is somewhat rigid to protect the soft tissue repair. The MTP joint is splinted in plantarflexion and slight varus for medial sesamoidectomy or valgus for lateral sesamoidectomy. After medial sesamoidectomy, patients may bear weight as tolerated in a protective boot or hard-soled shoe. The patient should wear a removable bunion splint for up to 6 weeks postoperatively. Because of the plantar incision itself, patients who undergo a lateral sesamoidectomy need to remain non–weight bearing (or heel touch-down weight bearing) for approximately 2 weeks. Thereafter, weight bearing is initiated, but the sutures remain in place for 3 or 4 weeks. The patient advances to hard-soled shoes beginning at about 6 weeks, and athletes should consider the incorporation of a turf toe plate in their shoe.

Various authors have reported on the results of sesamoidectomy. Inge and Ferguson,[23] in 1933, reviewed 41 feet with 25 having both sesamoids excised. Their study reported 42% of patients obtained complete relief, with some relief noted in 82% of patients who had a single sesamoid excised and in 64% of patients who had both excised. Leventen[24] found complete satisfaction in 18 of 23 sesamoidectomies. Mann and colleagues[25] reported on 21 sesamoidectomies. Nineteen patients in this series improved, but only 50% had complete relief, and full range of motion remained in only 66%. One of 13 patients who had a medial sesamoidectomy developed hallux valgus, and one of eight patients who had lateral sesamoidectomy developed hallux varus. Twelve patients developed toe flexion or push-off weakness.

SUMMARY

Turf toe injuries and sesamoid injuries are challenging because of the variety of causes that exist as sources of pain. Through a systematic approach to evaluation, injuries to the hallux MTP joint can be diagnosed properly, leading to accurate and efficient treatment. If conservative measures fail, operative interventions are available to relieve pain and restore function. With careful surgical technique and appropriate postoperative management, athletes can return to play and efficiently reach their preinjury level of participation.

REFERENCES

1. Clanton TO, Ford JJ. Turf toe injury. Clin Sports Med 1994;13(4):731–41.
2. Stokes IA, Hutton WC, Stott JR, et al. Forces under the hallux valgus foot before and after surgery. Clin Orthop Relat Res 1979;142:64–72.
3. Nigg BM. Biomechanical aspects of running. In: Nigg BM, editor. Biomechanics of running shoes. Champaign (IL): Human Kinetics Publishers; 1986. p. 1–25.
4. Bowers KD Jr, Martin RB. Turf-toe: a shoe-surface related football injury. Med Sci Sports 1976;8(2):81–3.
5. Coker TP, Arnold JA, Weber DL. Traumatic lesions of the metatarsophalangeal joint of the great toe in athletes. J Ark Med Soc 1978;74(8):309–17.
6. Clanton TO, Butler JE, Eggert A. Injuries to the metatarsophalangeal joints in athletes. Foot Ankle 1986;7(3):162–76.
7. Rodeo SA, O'Brien S, Warren RF, et al. Turf-toe: an analysis of metatarsophalangeal joint sprains in professional football players. Am J Sports Med 1990;18(3):280–5.
8. Watson TS, Anderson RB, Davis WH. Periarticular injuries to the hallux metatarsophalangeal joint in athletes. Foot Ankle Clin 2000;5(3):687–713.

9. Douglas DP, Davidson DM, Robinson JE, et al. Rupture of the medial collateral ligament of the first metatarsophalangeal joint in a professional soccer player. J Foot Ankle Surg 1997;36(5):388–90.

10. Prieskorn D, Graves SC, Smith RA. Morphometric analysis of the plantar plate apparatus of the first metatarsophalangeal joint. Foot Ankle 1993;14(4):204–7.

11. Tewes DP, Fischer DA, Fritts HM, et al. MRI findings of acute turf toe. A case report and review of anatomy. Clin Orthop Relat Res 1994;304:200–3.

12. Anderson RB. Turf toe injuries of the hallux metatarsophalangeal joint. Tech Foot Ankle Surg 2002;1(2):102–11.

13. Coughlin MJ. Sesamoid pain: causes and surgical treatment. Instr Course Lect 1990;39:23–5.

14. McBryde AM Jr, Anderson RB. Sesamoid foot problems in the athlete. Clin Sports Med 1998;7(1):51–60.

15. Jahss MH. The sesamoids of the hallux. Clin Orthop Relat Res 1981;157:88–97.

16. Rowe MM. Osteomyelitis of metatarsal sesamoid. Br Med J 1963;1(5337):1071–2.

17. Manoli A 2nd, Graham B. The subtle cavus foot, "the underpronator." Foot Ankle Int 2005;26(3):256–63.

18. Zinman H, Keret D, Reis ND. Fracture of the medial sesamoid bone of the hallux. J Trauma 1981;21(7):581–2.

19. Riley J, Seiner M. Internal fixation of a displaced tibial sesamoid fracture. J Am Podiatr Med Assoc 2001;91(10):536–9.

20. Anderson RB, McBryde AM Jr. Autogenous bone grafting of hallux sesamoid nonunions. Foot Ankle Int 1997;18(5):293–6.

21. Aper RL, Saltzman CL, Brown TD. The effect of hallux sesamoid resection on the effective moment of the flexor hallucis brevis. Foot Ankle Int 1994;15(9):462–70.

22. Aper RL, Saltzman CL, Brown TD. The effect of hallux sesamoid excision on the flexor hallucis longus moment arm. Clin Orthop Relat Res 1996;325:209–17.

23. Inge GAL, Ferguson AB. Surgery of the sesamoid bones of the great toe. Arch Surg 1933;27:466–89.

24. Leventen EO. Sesamoid disorders and treatment. An update. Clin Orthop Relat Res 1991;269:236–40.

25. Mann RA, Coughlin MJ, Baxter D, et al. Sesamoidectomy of the great toe. Presented at the 15th Annual American Orthopaedic Foot and Ankle Society Meeting. Las Vegas: January 24,1985.

The Complicated Jones Fracture, Including Revision and Malalignment

Angus M. McBryde, Jr, MD[a,b,*]

KEYWORDS

- Jones fracture • Base fifth metatarsal fracture • Decayed
- Nonunion • Fixation devices • Complications

The "Jones fracture" as presented (December 19, 1901) and later described by Liverpool surgeon Robert Jones[1,2] is the first of the three fracture types that occur at the base of the fifth metatarsal. The first is an acute fracture, which can be comminuted, or an avulsion-type involving the tuberosity itself. The second is the true "Jones fracture." Usually a transverse injury, it involves the fourth and fifth intermetatarsal facets on the medial side[3] and the metaphyseal junction. The Jones fracture occurs in an area between the tuberosity fractures and the stress fracture (**Fig. 1**). The third is a stress fracture involving the proximal diaphysis.[4]

For this article, radiographs were culled over a 33-month period at the outpatient Ankle and Foot Service of the Andrews Sports Medicine and Orthopaedic Center (ASMOC) in Birmingham, Alabama. There were 170 base fifth metatarsal fractures found. Bone fractures of the fifth metatarsal occur commonly in an active or athletic population. Unlike the distal fifth metatarsal fractures in elite athletes who can often be treated nonoperatively, the proximal fractures are best treated by internal fixation.[5] Fractures of the base of the fifth metatarsal cause significant functional disability in all ages and with all work-related, recreational, and competitive activities. Chasing and obtaining union can be difficult and is only exceeded by the difficulty maintaining that union and preventing refracture (**Figs. 2** and **3**). Stewart[6] in 1960 and Dameron[7] in 1975 originally called attention to the problem. Anderson[8] in 1976, on the contrary, continued to find no problem gaining base fifth metatarsal union. In 1979, Zelko and colleagues[9] documented proximal diaphyseal problems. In 1984, Torg and colleagues[10] classified or described: (1) an acute fracture, (2) delayed union, and (3) nonunion.

[a] Andrews Sports Medicine & Orthopaedic Center, Birmingham, AL, USA
[b] American Sports Medicine Institute, 2660 10th Avenue, South, Suite 505, Birmingham, AL 35205, USA
* American Sports Medicine Institute, 2660 10th Avenue, South, Suite 505, Birmingham, AL 35205.
E-mail address: mcbrydea@aol.com

Foot Ankle Clin N Am 14 (2009) 151–168
doi:10.1016/j.fcl.2009.04.001
1083-7515/09/$ – see front matter © 2009 Elsevier Inc. All rights reserved.

foot.theclinics.com

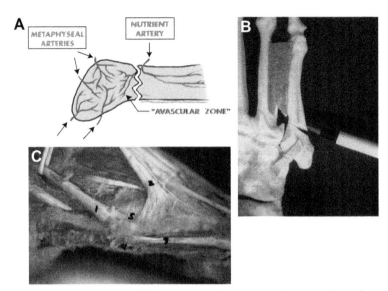

Fig. 1. (A) Vascular anatomy base fifth. (*From* Smith JW, Arnoczky SP, Hersh A. The intraosseous blood supply of the fifth metatarsal: implications for proximal fracture healing. Foot Ankle 1992;13:144; with permission.) (B) Approximate position of Jones fracture. (C) Cadaver anatomy with peroneus brevis 1, peroneus tertius 2, abductor digiti minimi 3, plantar aponeurosis lateral aspect 4, base fifth metatarsal 5. (*From* McBryde AM and Barfield WR. Stress fractures of the foot and ankle. Foot and Ankle Clinics 1999;4(4):900; with permission.)

Byrd[11] described the probable mechanics involved. He also reviewed the original described Jones fracture and noted the probability of it being a stress fracture.

Forty-five percent of children's metatarsal fractures involve the base of the fifth metatarsal. For the most part, the described five types of fifth metatarsal base fractures in children can be treated in a similar way to the comparable adult fractures.[12] Iselin's disease uniquely can give base fifth metatarsal problems when apophyseal partial or complete avulsions happen.

Significant progress has been made in understanding these fractures and the surrounding issues. Targeted anatomy and biomechanics, the operative devices available, and rehabilitation programs including orthoses[13] have helped project and plan for early union, early weight bearing, and the minimization of complications. Even so, studies continue to show substantial morbidity—especially in the competitive or recreational athletic population and in the "physically" working population.

TREATMENT PROTOCOL AND OPTIONS

In general, tuberosity fractures, acute Jones fractures, and diaphyseal stress fractures have specific anatomic localization.[3,14] Though numerous open and closed regimens have been advised, nonoperative treatment has traditionally been utilized. Literature over the last 35 years has increasingly noted that these fractures treated nonoperatively can fail to unite and have complications as outlined later.[15] Improved technique and technical advances enable high-performance athletes or leg-based workers to benefit from a more aggressive and usually surgical approach.

In 1992, Rettig and colleagues[16] described proximal fifth metatarsal fractures that are tuberosity fractures; that is, apophyseal avulsion fracture (Iselin's disease), styloid process fracture, metaphyseal fracture, and avulsion fracture. These fractures also must be respected and may need surgery (**Figs. 4** and **5**). When undisplaced, tuberosity fractures are traditionally treated casually[3] with an accommodative shoe, boot, or similar device. Weight bearing is allowed at 3 weeks post injury or even earlier. Slow healing can result. On the contrary, limited weight bearing and later mobilization should occur only when symptoms and tenderness abate and when imaging evidence of early union (3 to 4 weeks) is present. Problems, however, can occur.[16–18] This article does not explore tuberosity fractures in any depth (**Fig. 6**).

ANATOMY DESCRIPTION AND TYPE OF FRACTURE

Jones fracture has had various interpretations;[6] however, is universally defined as a skeletally mature injury without prior symptoms occurring at the metaphyseal diaphyseal junction of the fifth metatarsal base. Acute-on-chronic fracture[19] is equivalent to stress fracture when the proximal diaphyseal area is involved.[11,20]

The exact fracture position and diagnosis of transitional proximal diaphyseal fracture as stress fracture or Jones fracture is academic and is a matter of nomenclature. The important question is whether using one diagnos is instead of the other leads to a different outcome. Most studies do not differentiate.[21,22] There are no studies that offer a conclusive level of evidence either way. There is significant clinical discrepancy between these two entities. A stress fracture of the proximal diaphysis involves the proximal 1.5 cm of the metatarsal shaft or diaphysis, and a Jones fracture involves the metaphyseal–diaphyseal junction and, often, the metatarsal fourth-fifth proximal joint.[10,23] The issue remains controversial.[3] The characteristics of the two fractures differ in four respects:[24] Stress fractures can have (1) a history of symptoms prior to an acute event and no earlier known fracture, (2) physical exam compatibility (ie, palpable bump), (3) imaging callus or sclerosis indicating pre-event stress changes,[25] (4) open examination findings (in the rare case that open treatment is necessary).

Historically the Jones fracture has been treated with a short leg cast. Crutches are often necessary to alleviate symptoms. Transition to a walker boot follows with the same principle of keeping the level of leg-based activity below that which causes symptoms. Loss of fifth metatarsal tenderness and imaging evidence of healing must also be present before return to play or return to leg-based activity such as running, soccer, football, or dance. Discussion continues regarding the athlete and the nonathlete. A more aggressive approach of intramedullary fixation has evolved for the athlete to avoid prolonged healing.[21,26] The cannulated intramedullary screw (**Fig. 7**) has simplified both instrumentation and time requirements. Though this operative approach allows quicker return for the athlete, numerous complications and problems occur. On the other hand, the morbidity of redo operative procedures is rivaled by the often-delayed fixation procedures necessary after unsuccessful nonoperative treatment.[9]

Bone stimulation is used as an adjunct or as primary therapy in selected cases. It is frequently utilized in the secondary school, collegiate, and professional athletic population simply for its user-friendliness and its noninvasive requirements.[3,27,28] If union results, there can be an earlier return to play and avoidance of more costly surgery.

Studies by Shereff and colleagues,[29] and Smith and colleagues,[30] show a potential zone of intraosseous avascularity that may help explain proximal diaphyseal slow healing (see **Fig. 1**A). My personal feeling is that rates of union, refracture, and other indices (eg, imaging union, remodeling time) differ with the two types of fracture.[3,31,32] The clear implication is that Jones fracture and proximal diaphysis fifth-metatarsal

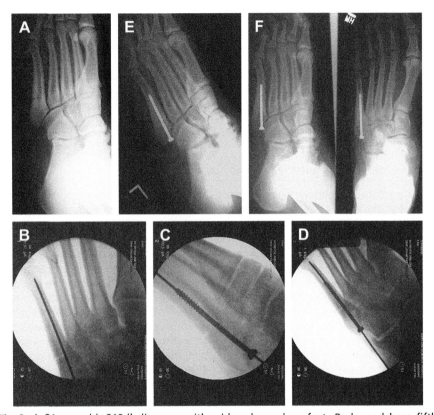

Fig. 2. A 21-year-old, 310-lb lineman with wide, planovalgus feet. Prolonged base fifth metatarsal problems effectively ended his football career. Imaging showed unequivocal standing anteroposterior evidence of fifth metatarsal offload laterally. Orthoses were never user-friendly. (*A*) 3/29/03 Initial injury and surgery. (*B*) 6/6/03 Fine line still present on radiograph 3 months postoperative. (*C*) 8/28/03 CT scan with nonunion and only partial peripheral union. (*D*) 12/23/03 Second surgery at 9 months with stainless steel 6.5-mm cannulated screw with intramedullary bone graft without complication. (*E*) 4/22/04 Complete healing radiographically at 4 months postoperative and no symptoms before early practice return. (*F*) 8/13/04 Symptoms with running in preparation for football. CT scan with plantar cortical infraction. (*G–J*) This was the effective end of his football career after 18 months of maximized treatment and rehabilitation.

stress fractures are two different entities.[24] Favorable outcomes depend on unique awareness of each during both acute care and rehabilitation management.

Most base fifth metatarsal fractures are seen by or referred to orthopedists.[32] However, primary care or sports medicine physicians handle many of these fractures initially. At the ASMOC clinic, approximately 50% are primary-care treated or triaged for surgery early or late in the process.

Predisposing factors on which to base diagnosis of fifth metatarsal injuries include:

Varus hindfoot.
Raikin and colleagues[13] noted that 18 of 20 patients with Jones fractures had clinical or radiographic rearfoot varus in keeping with previous observations.[7,24,33] A nonoperative or postoperative lateral heel or sole wedge can

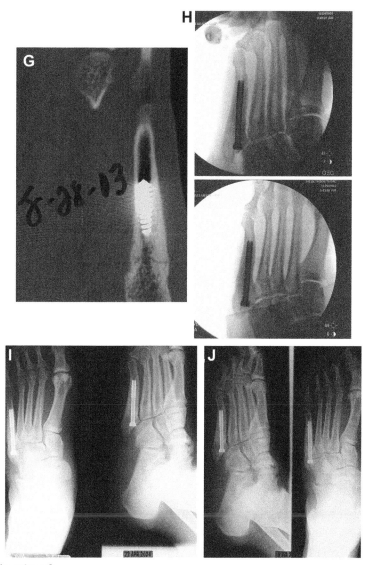

Fig. 2. (*continued*)

be helpful and should routinely be used in athletes with varus heels. For recurrent inversion sprain or chronic related foot plant problems, a lateralizing calcaneal osteotomy or Dwyer lateral closing wedge osteotomy are considerations.

Old fracture with a new refracture.

There is no appropriate classification for these refractures. Eventual union can require cessation of the inciting activity or sport (**Fig. 8**). Lack of correction of the biomechanical abnormality, early removal of a screw, inadequate rehabilitation, including a poorly constructed home exercise program, can lead to refracture or delayed healing.

Tight plantar aponeurosis and short peroneal muscle length and excursion.[34–36]

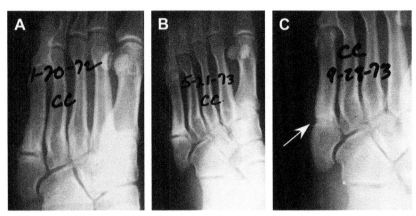

Fig. 3. A 25-year-old Australian Olympic basketball player and coach with longstanding nonunion. (*A*) Apparent union of a known stress fracture in basketball preseason and playing with increasing pain early season. (*B*) "Played hurt" all season. (*C*) United at 1 year.

> Peroneal weakness relative to the posterior tibial strength is often present, especially with a history of ankle sprain, and is a common predisposing factor in lateral foot overload and delayed union or refracture.

PROBLEMS AND COMPLICATIONS WITH THE TREATMENT OF JONES FRACTURES

Intramedullary screw fixation, whether initially or with a nonunion or refracture, is the procedure of choice.[25,32–43] Nunley and Glisson[44] use open reduction and internal fixation in young athletic patients with excellent results. Zogby and Baker,[45] and Acker and Drez[46] still champion nonoperative or individual treatment in active people.

Proper Diagnosis

The history, the leg-ankle-foot examination, and imaging are important. Steroid or nonsteroidal differential diagnostic injection can help (ie, peroneal avulsion or related-injury question) lateral column Lisfranc sprain, and stress inversion for displacement or stability.

Imaging

Imaging should include anteroposterior standing and lateral standing views of both feet plus an oblique view of the foot or base fifth metatarsal.[47] MRI, limited bone scan, and CT scan (see **Figs. 2C and 9C**) with one to two millimeter cuts are helpful with equivocal injury, suspected associated injury, and later stages of treatment and management with questionable union or nonunion.

Device Selection and Use

Selection and use of devices used in treatment of Jones fractures include:

Cannulated (see **Fig. 7**) and solid screw systems[43,48] (ByrdT, personal communication, 1990) are currently accepted as the best fixation.[48–51] These screws, when implanted properly, provide for bending and tension stability. There seems to be less resistance to torsional stress.[41] Cost must always be a consideration.
The Herbert-Whipple screw[52] is occasionally used.
Titanium screws have a modulus of elasticity that more closely resembles cortical bone than do stainless steel screws.[35] This provides some rationale for their use.

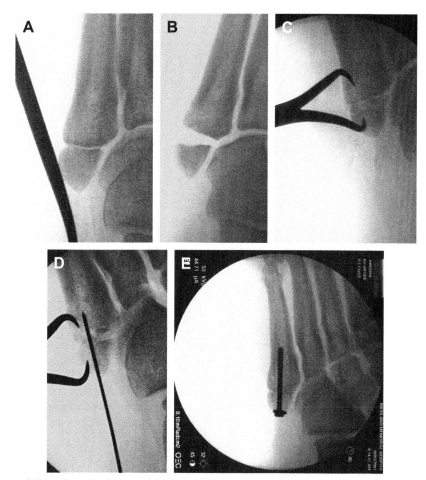

Fig. 4. (*A*) A tuberosity fracture into cuboid fifth metatarsal joint. (*B*) Original fracture with size and displacement "borderline Jones" but requiring decision making between open reduction with internal fixation and excision. Examination under anesthesia shows (*C*) significant displacement, (*D*) reduction, and (*E*) fixation with a smaller cannulated screw (4.0 mm) for a smaller fragment; including a washer.

> They can be difficult to remove if they ever break because they adhere to the surrounding bone.
>
> Headless, tapered, and variable pitch screws offer no more than 6.5mm partially threaded cancellous lag screws.[53]
>
> Small plates destroy extraosseous blood supply, which is important because intraosseous blood supply has been unequivocally damaged. The occasional use of small plates may be necessary as in certain types of comminution. These are rarely used in the athlete.

Screw Size

Screw size selection is essential. Preoperative templates with current computer graphics (measurement and orientation) are available, easy, and essential for measuring canal width at three points. Correct angulation and rotation of the shaft

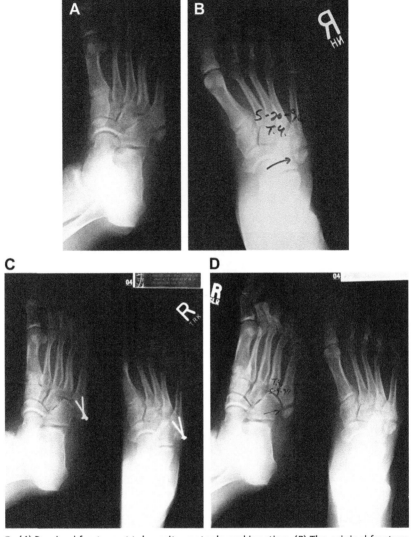

Fig. 5. (A) Proximal fracture at tuberosity–metaphyseal junction. (B) The original fracture. (C) Two screws were placed with ongoing pain and limp coupled with boot and non-weight bearing. (D) Nonunion with continued pain. At 1 year, metal was removed, the fragment excised, and peroneus brevis reattached. Running at 4 months with no pain.

is important. Mini C-arm superimposition with the screw is easy to do and provides a predictable fit and fill. It is important to use the largest screw that is practical even though there is some evidence that with three-point bending failure loads have little variation.[54] Less than a 4-mm screw diameter is not recommended except in certain circumstances (eg, children and unusually sized adult bones[55]). Lag screw length is important.[56] Optional use of a washer in selected cases can be appropriate (see **Fig. 4**C) or inappropriate (see **Fig. 6**). Position the screw so it stays intramedullary. An intramedullary screw perpendicular to the fracture is recommended in nontuberosity fractures.[56] Large body mass (usually in the athlete) requires a large screw (5.5 or

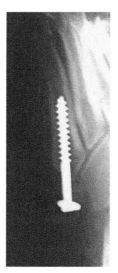

Fig. 6. Poor decision making and poor technique can create major problems. A washer and a long, oversized screw failed in this attempt to reduce a small tuberosity fragment. Extrication of metal and excision of the fragment followed with difficulty.

6.5) and protected early return. Since the screw should remain in place indefinitely, proper placement is necessary. The screw should not involve the cuboid or fourth-fifth metatarsal joint.

Biologics

Adjunctive biologic IGNITE (Wright Medical Technology, Inc., Arlington, TN, USA) (**Fig. 9**) or other biologics (including autogenous bone graft) can and should be used for Jones fracture nonunion,[57] especially when other comorbidities that can prevent union are present (eg, weight, wide splayfoot, smoking, diabetes).

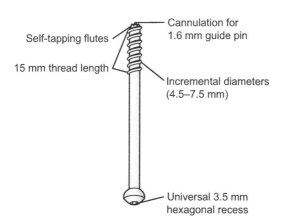

Fig. 7. Numerous screws are usable for fifth metatarsal. Here is general construct of a cannulated screw that can be used for this fracture.

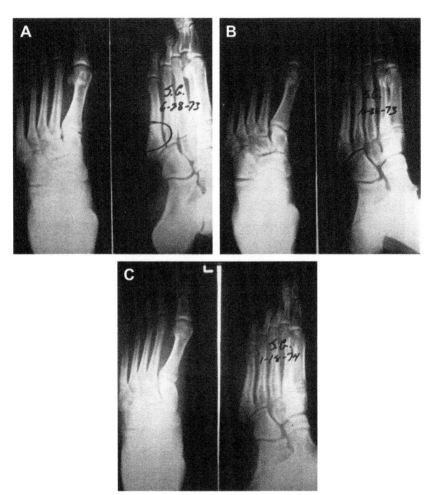

Fig. 8. A 20- year-old basketball player with spring-summer camp pain leading to stress fracture of the proximal diaphysis of the fifth metatarsal. (*A*) At the time of injury. (*B*) Completion of the fracture radiographically 4 months after presentation, including 6 weeks of casting. (*C*) Early obscuring of the fracture site 6.5 months after presentation. (*From* McBryde AM Jr. Stress fractures. In: Baxter DE, editor. The foot and ankle in sport. 1st edition. Mosby; 1995. p. 87; with permission.)

Patient Compliance

Weight bearing should not occur (at the earliest) until 3 weeks after injury. Even then, there must be partial weight bearing if full weight bearing is painful. The results of patient noncompliance are seen in **Fig. 10**.

Exogenous Factors

Smoking, systemic steroid dosages, or other factors that induce osteoporosis are deterrents to union and should be corrected when possible. Types 1 and 2 diabetes can create potential morbidity.[58]

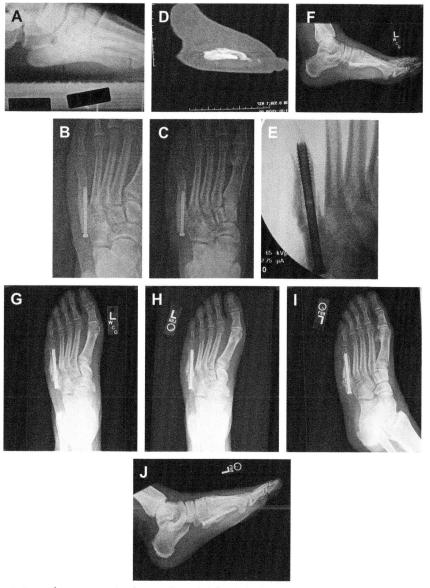

Fig. 9. Jones fracture proximal metaphyseal. (*A*) Original injury and surgery. (*B*) Early union at 2 months; but with acute insecurity with an event while on a treadmill 8 weeks postoperative with probable refracture. (*C*) Refusion with IGNITE (biologic) and larger 6.5 screw. (*D*) Early union at 5 months after second surgery. (*E–J*) Varying views. (*Courtesy of* Bob Anderson, MD, Charlotte, NC).

Joint Involvement

Calcaneocuboid and cuboid-metatarsal joint, or other bony involvement with significant displacement, needs occasional specifically directed operative attention. The secondary rehabilitation attention to soft tissue and joint mobilization may need modification.

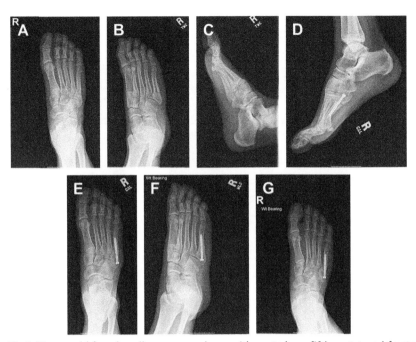

Fig. 10. A 23-year-old female college soccer player with acute base fifth metatarsal fracture. (A) Noncompliance and too much loading early caused delayed union and retreatment. (B) 4/19/08 Injury on the soccer field. (C) 4/24/08 5.0-mm titanium cannulated screw placed. (D) 5/19/08 Cast removed. Transitioned to Cam walker boot use. Activity not athletic, but much walking caused rotation. (E–G) 7/25/08 No symptoms but radiograph evidence of plantar lateral gapping. 9/14/08 Flag football injury and Cam boot replaced. 11/24/08 No tenderness but still in a boot and treatment ongoing for 7-plus months.

Soft-tissue Attachment Involvement

Peroneal tendon insertion and other soft-tissue attachment involvement must be considered preoperatively and addressed if major tears are present. MRI is appropriate in this circumstance. Rehabilitation issues such as tendency to recurrence and mechanical offloading can be secondarily affected.

Sural or Other Nerve Injury

Avoid nerve injury by meticulous dissection. Loupes are ideal especially if there is an open component to any portion of the reduction and fixation.[59]

Judgment and Surgical Technique Points

Key points in judgment and surgical technique include:[60]

  Anatomic knowledge. Surgical ability to "travel around" the lateral column or midfoot.
  A drill guide or sleeve should be used with care to avoid skin pressure and provide tissue protection.
  Tissue protection is mandatory to prevent skin and soft tissue-pressure necrosis, which can be unnoticed initially.

Power drills and drill bits can quickly produce thermal necrosis of bone and/or soft tissue. Saline, frequent few second rests, mineral oil, graduated drill size (if not cannulated) are all facilitators of screw placement.

Functional orthotic management plus shoe modification should be considered in at-risk athletes for the first 6 to 12 months after union. Characteristics of certain athletes make them at risk for refracture. Cavus feet, a large frame coupled with a wide pronated foot, a shoe size of 13 and higher, a prior similar fracture, and fracture displacement are risk factors. Semirigid orthoses with cushion and control should be supplemented by a circumscribed, less dense compound to further unload the base and head of the fifth metatarsal. Lateral column posting at the forefoot and hindfoot can be preventive in the varus rearfoot.

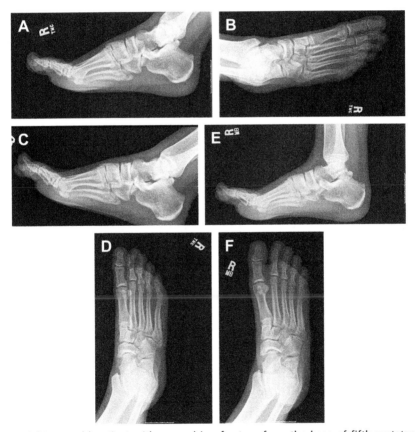

Fig. 11. A 21-year-old patient with an avulsion fracture from the base of fifth metatarsal, surgery with excision of the fragment and reattachment using #2 OrthoCord, drill holes, and reattachment. Four months later, he was healed and playing ball with mild pain. Orthoses were used to unload the fifth metatarsal. (A) 11/29/06 Presents with 3-week history of pain with running. Cam walker boot and bone stimulation were initial treatment. (B) 6/6/07 Improved but still symptomatic. (C) 9/18/07 Base fifth metatarsal with no symptoms. (D–F) MRI showed an os trigonum with posterior edema and accessory navicular along with much increased signal at the base of the fifth metatarsal. Injuries cluster.

Rehabilitation

A longer non–weight-bearing time is required with a nonoperative approach.[61] The biomechanics of the lateral midfoot may be changed if there has been a preexisting or injury-related difference in strength status locally. Attachment to the base of the fifth metatarsal relative to the peroneus brevis, the peroneus tertius, the plantar aponeurotic ligament (plantar fascia), or the abductor digiti quinti may create deranged biomechanics. This can be suspected early on[62] and may have been involved with the index injury or even the subsequent surgery (**Fig. 11**). These changed biomechanics may thus prevent unloading or, in fact, may precipitate overload of the base of the fifth metatarsal.

The increased medial column arch support—as occurs with off-the-shelf orthoses—can cause lateral overload.[63] Guettler and colleagues,[64] however, noted reduced stresses beneath the fifth metatarsal using an orthosis with a significant arch support. The fifth metatarsal base/head certainly can be pushed further off the shoe sole in the splayfoot or wide foot. The peroneals eccentrically try to stabilize the foot in the shoe. Pes planus, wide-splayed feet, and varus thrust can cause this foot shift with lateral column overload. This can leave the midfoot and forefoot relatively unsupported or actually produce complete lateral foot-plant offload.

Premature Return to Play

Criteria should progressively include:

No tenderness
Imaging evidence of union

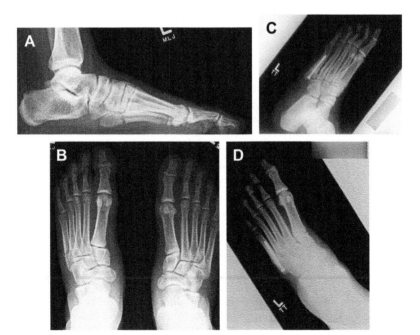

Fig. 12. A 22-year-old college lineman. No MRI necessary. Proximal diaphyseal fracture. *(A)* Lateral *(B)* Anterior-posterior *(C)* 8-2-08 Surgery *(D)* Union using a 5.0mm titanium cannulated screw. Available for fall football at approximately 4 weeks postoperative. No sequelae.

Regaining of strength through eccentric and concentric open-chain or muscle-specific work

Closed chain nonimpact activities such as cycling, elliptical, or similar equipment

Graduated return to impact loading

Sport-specific agility work.

ADJUNCTIVE POSTOPERATIVE COURSE REHABILITATION

The key to nonoperative or operative success and return to play is rehabilitation (**Fig. 12**). Rehabilitation is a combination of compliance, formal or informal protocol, and avoidance of single or repetitive stress overload until union is unequivocal on imaging, symptoms are absent clinically, and strength and function are fully restored.

A soft-tissue Jones dressing was found to work better than a cast for immediate postoperative immobilization with 92 "excellent" compared to 86 "good" results. Recuperation in 33 days compared to 46 days occurred with this approach.[65] A trilaminar splint including a sugar tong and a posterior component would seem more appropriate. Deep-water running for lower-trunk or extremity injury can be very helpful.[66] The level of pain dictates the activity during rehabilitation. Any activity that causes foot-related pain is unacceptable; any pain-free activity is allowed. Cycling upright or recumbent at 3 to 4 weeks can be started. Early on, linear running should not be too slow. Sprinting can begin when all nonagility leg-based work, such as cycling, has proved doable and progressive.

SUMMARY

The treatment of fractures of the base of the fifth metatarsal and specifically the non-tuberosity Jones fracture has evolved from a casual and limited nonoperative approach to a much more aggressive and operative framework. Although the nonoperative approach remains viable, reliable, and accepted, the exigencies and desires of the active population—particularly the athletic and leg-based working population—requires sooner-rather-than-later return to play or work. Fortunately, these needs can be matched by the available and functioning orthopedic practice of intramedullary screw fixation. This practice is coupled with prevention, recognition (ie, varus), reliable orthopedic techniques, the orthopedist's surgical skills, and developed devices (ie, intramedullary screw fixation systems) necessary for successful surgery. However, there continue to be pitfalls in surgical and rehabilitation management that lead to complications. Recent attention directed toward handling those complications promise better, quicker, and more reliable return to play or to work for the patient.

REFERENCES

1. Browne E, Jones R. Fracture of the fifth metatarsal bone summary. In: Liverpool Medico-Chirurgical, Series of Foreign Books. Proceedings of the Fifth Ordinary Meeting. Liverpool: 1901. p. 103–11.
2. Jones R. Fracture of the base of the fifth metatarsal bone by indirect violence. Ann Surg 1902;XXXV:697–700.
3. Rosenberg GA, Sferra JJ. Treatment strategies for acute fractures and nonunions of the proximal fifth metatarsal. J Am Acad Orthop Surg 2000;8(5):332–8.
4. DeLee JC. Stress fractures of the base of the fifth metatarsal, distal to the tuberosity. Presentation at the American Orthopaedic Society for Sports Medicine Annual Meeting, July 6–9,1986. Sun Valley, Idaho.

5. O'Malley MJ, Hamilton WG, Munyak J, et al. "Dancer's fracture." Am J Sports Med 1996;24(2):240–3.
6. Stewart M. Jones's fracture: fracture of the base of fifth metatarsal. Clin Orthop 1960;16:190–8.
7. Dameron T. Fractures and anatomical variations of the proximal portion of the fifth metatarsal. J Bone Joint Surg Am 1975;57(6):788–92.
8. Anderson LD. Injuries of the forefoot; fracture of the base of the fifth metatarsal. Clin Orthop Relat Res 1977;122:18–27.
9. Zelko R, Torg J, Rachun A. Proximal diaphyseal fractures of the fifth metatarsal—treatment of the fractures and their complications in athletes. Am J Sports Med 1979;7(2):95–101.
10. Torg J, Balduini F, Zelko R, et al. Fractures of the base of the fifth metatarsal distal to the tuberosity. J Bone Joint Surg Am 1984;66(2):209–14.
11. Byrd T. Jones fracture: relearning an old injury. South Med J 1992;85(7):748–50.
12. Herrera-Soto JA, Scherb M, Duffy MF, et al. Fractures of the fifth metatarsal in children and adolescents. J Pediatr Orthop 2007;27(4):427–31.
13. Raikin SM, Slenker N, Ratigan B. The association of a varus hindfoot and fracture of the fifth metatarsal metaphyseal-diaphyseal junction. Am J Sports Med 2008; 36(7):1367–72.
14. McBryde AM. Stress fractures in athletes. Am J Sports Med 1975;3:212–7.
15. Chuckpaiwong B, Queen RM, Easley ME, et al. Distinguishing Jones and proximal diaphyseal fractures of the fifth metatarsal. Clin Orthop Relat Res 2008; 466:1966–70.
16. Rettig A, Shelbourne KD, Wilckens J. The surgical treatment of symptomatic nonunions of the proximal metaphyseal fifth metatarsal in athletes. Am J Sports Med 1992;20(1):50–4.
17. Husain ZS, DeFronzo DJ. Relative stability of tension band vs. two-cortex screw fixation for treating fifth metatarsal base avulsion fractures. J Foot Ankle Surg 2000;39(2):89–95.
18. Egol K, Walsh M, Rosenblatt K, et al. Avulsion fractures of the fifth metatarsal base: a prospective outcome study. Foot Ankle Int 2007;28(2):581–3.
19. Yu W, Shapiro M. Fractures of the fifth metatarsal: careful identification for optimal treatment. Phys and Sports Med 1998;26(2):47–64.
20. McBryde AM. Stress fractures in runners. In: D'Ambrosia R, Drez D, editors. Prevention and treatment of running injuries. Thorofare (NJ): Slack Inc.; 1989. p. 50–77.
21. Arangio G. Proximal diaphyseal fractures of the fifth metatarsal (Jones' fracture): two cases treated by cross-pinning with review of 106 cases. Foot Ankle 1983; 3(5):293–6.
22. Glasgow MD, Naranja RJ, Glasgow S, et al. Analysis of failed surgical management of fractures of the base of the fifth metatarsal distal to the tuberosity: the Jones fracture. Foot Ankle Int 1996;17(8):449–57.
23. McBryde AM Jr. Stress fractures. In: Baxter DE, editor. The foot and ankle in sport [First edition]. Saunders; 1995. p. 81–93.
24. DeLee J, Evans P, Julian J. Stress fracture of the fifth metatarsal. Am J Sports Med 1983;11(5):349–53.
25. Rehman S, Kashyap S. Proximal fifth metatarsal stress fracture treated by early open reduction and internal fixation. Orthopedics 2004;27(11):1196–8.
26. Sammarco GJ, Carrasquillo HA. Intramedullary fixation of metatarsal fracture and nonunion. Two methods of treatment. Orthop Clin North Am 1995;26(2): 265–72.

27. Holmes GV. Treatment of delayed unions and nonunions of the proximal fifth metatarsal with pulsed electromagnetic fields. Foot Ankle Int 1994;15(10):552–6.
28. McBryde AM, Barfield WR. Stress fractures of the foot and ankle, foot and ankle. Foot Ankle Clin 1999;4(4):881–909.
29. Shereff M, Yang Q, Kummer F, et al. Vascular anatomy of the fifth metatarsal. Foot Ankle 1991;11(6):350–3, Cite for figure.
30. Smith J, Arnoczky S, Hersh A. The intraosseous blood supply of the fifth metatarsal: implications for proximal fracture healing. Am Ortho Foot Society, Inc. Foot Ankle 1992;13(3):143–52.
31. Dameron T. Fractures of the proximal fifth metatarsal: selecting the best treatment option. J Am Acad Orthop Surg 1995;3(2):110–4.
32. Strayer SM, Reece SG, Petrizzi MJ. Fractures of the proximal fifth metatarsal. Am Fam Physician 1999;(May):1–9.
33. Sammarco GJ. Be alert for Jones fractures. Phys and Spts Med 1992;20(6):101–10.
34. Fairen M, Guillen J, Busto J, et al. Fractures of the fifth metatarsal in basketball players. Knee Surg Sports Traumatol Arthrosc 1999;7:373–7.
35. Lawrence SJ, Botte MJ. Jones' fractures and related fractures of the proximal fifth metatarsal. Foot Ankle 1993;14(6):358–65.
36. Theodorou D, Theodorou S, Kakitsubata Y, et al. Fractures of proximal portion of fifth metatarsal bone: anatomic and imaging evidence of a pathogenesis of avulsion of the plantar aponeurosis and the short peroneal muscle tendon. Radiology 2003;226(3):857–65.
37. Larson CM, Almedinders LC, Taft TM, et al. Intramedullary screw fixation of Jones fractures. Am J Sports Med 2002;30(1):55–60.
38. Wright RW, Fischer DA, Shively RA, et al. Refracture of proximal fifth metatarsal (Jones) fracture after intramedullary screw fixation in athletes. Am J Sports Med 2000;28(5):732–6.
39. Mindrebo N, Shelbourne KD, Van Meter CD, et al. Outpatient percutaneous screw fixation of the acute Jones fracture. Am J Sports Med 1993;21(5):720–3.
40. Porter DA, Duncan M, Meyer S. Fifth metatarsal Jones fracture fixation with a 4.5-mm cannulated stainless steel screw in the competitive and recreational athlete. Am J Sports Med 2005;33(5):726–33.
41. Vertullo CJ, Glisson RR, Nunley JA. Torsional strains in the proximal fifth metatarsal: implications for Jones and stress fracture management. Foot Ankle Int 2004;25(9):650–6.
42. Kavanaugh JH, Brower TD, Mann RV. The Jones fracture revisited. J Bone Joint Surg Am 1978;60(6):776–82.
43. Nunley JA, Glisson RR. A new option for intramedullary fixation of Jones fractures: the Charlotte Carolina Jones fracture system. Foot Ankle Int 2008;29(12):1216–21.
44. Nunley JA. Fractures of the base of the fifth metatarsal: the Jones fracture. Orthop Clin North Am 2001;32(1):171–80.
45. Zogby R, Baker B. A review of nonoperative treatment of Jones' fracture. Am J Sports Med 1987;15(4):304–7.
46. Acker JH, Drez D. Nonoperative treatment of stress fractures of the proximal shaft of the fifth metatarsal (Jones' fracture). Foot Ankle 1986;7(3):152–5.
47. Pao DG, Keats TE, Dussault RG. Avulsion fracture of the base of the fifth metatarsal not seen on conventional radiography of the foot: the need for an additional projection. AJR Am J Roentgenol 2000;175:549–52.
48. Retief C, Stuck R, Sartori M, et al. Fifth metatarsal base fracture distal to the tuberosity: the Jones fracture—comparing Kirschner wire-tension band and ao

malleolar screw fixation [annual]. Loyola University Chicago. Orthopaedic Journal 1998;VIII:56–60.

49. Noblin DJ, Low K, Browne JE, et al. Jones fractures in the elite football player. J Surg Orthop Adv 2004;13(3):156–60.
50. Clapper MF, O'Brien TJ, Lyons PM. Fractures of the fifth metatarsal: analysis of a fracture registry. Clin Orthop Relat Res 1995;315:238–41.
51. Portland G, Kelikian A, Kodros S. Acute surgical management of Jones' fractures. Foot Ankle Int 2003;24(11):829–33.
52. Reimer H, Kreibich M, Konigstein R, et al. Expanded indications for the Herbert-screw osteosynthesis. Unfallchirurgie 1995;21(5):251–9.
53. Sides SD, Fetter NL, Glisson BS, et al. Bending stiffness and pull-out strength of tapered, variable pitch screws, and 6.5mm cancellous screws in acute Jones fractures. Foot Ankle Int 2006;27(10):821–5.
54. Shah SN, Knoblich GO, Lindsey DP, et al. Intramedullary screw fixation of proximal fifth metatarsal fractures: a biomechanical study. Foot Ankle Int 2001;22(7):581–4.
55. Reese K, Litsky A, Kaeding C, et al. Cannulated screw fixation of Jones fractures: a clinical and biomechanical study. Am J Sports Med 2004;32(7):1736–42.
56. Moshirfar A, Campbell J, Molloy S, et al. Fifth metatarsal tuberosity fracture fixation: a biomechanical study. Foot Ankle Int 2003;24(8):630–3.
57. Mologne TS, Lundeen JM, Clapper MF, et al. Early screw fixation versus casting in the treatment of acute Jones fractures. Am J Sports Med 2005;33(7):970–5.
58. Yue JJ, Marcus RE. The role of internal fixation in the treatment of Jones fractures in diabetics. Foot Ankle Int 1996;17(9):559–62.
59. Donley B, McCollum M, Murphy A. Risk of sural nerve injury with intramedullary screw fixation of fifth metatarsal fractures: a cadaver study. Foot Ankle Int 1999;20(3):182–4.
60. Nunley JA. Jones fracture technique. Tech Foot Ankle Surg 2002;1(2):131–7.
61. Vorlat P, Achtergael W, Haentjens P. Predictors of outcome of non-displaced fractures of the base of the fifth metatarsal. (SICOT). Int Orthop 2007;31:5–10.
62. Carp L. Fracture of the fifth metatarsal bone, with special reference to delayed union. Ann Surg 1927;308–20.
63. Yu B, Preston J, Queen R, et al. Effects of wearing foot orthosis with medial arch support on the fifth metatarsal loading and ankle inversion angle in selected basketball tasks. J Orthop Sports Phys Ther 2007;37(4):186–91.
64. Guettler J, Ruskan G, Bytomski J, et al. Fifth metatarsal stress fractures in elite basketball players: evaluation of forces acting on the fifth metatarsal. Am J Orthop 2006;532–6.
65. Wiener BD, Linder JF, Giattini JF. Treatment of fractures of the fifth metatarsal: a prospective study. Foot Ankle Int 1997;18(5):267–9.
66. Frangolias DD, Taunton JE, Rhodes EC, et al. Maintenance of aerobic capacity during recovery from right foot Jones fracture: a case report. Clin J Sport Med 1997;7(1):54–8.

Lisfranc Injuries in Sport

Matthew DeOrio, MD[a], Melissa Erickson, MD[b],
Federico Giuseppe Usuelli, MD[c], Mark Easley, MD[d],*

KEYWORDS

• Midfoot sprain • Lisfranc ligament • Sports injuries

The Lisfranc joint complex is composed of the articulation between the midfoot and forefoot. The joint is named after Jacques Lisfranc de Saint-Martin (1787–1847), a French army field surgeon who described amputation through the tarsometatarsal (TMT) joint, yet did not describe the mechanism of injury or the importance of anatomic reduction following the injury.[1,2] Lisfranc injuries have traditionally been associated with high-energy trauma such as motor vehicle collisions and industrial accidents.[3,4] Recently, there has been a greater appreciation of midfoot sprains that represent a spectrum of injury to the Lisfranc ligament complex.[5] As a result, there has been an increased incidence of such injury resulting from low-energy trauma in activities ranging from recreational activity to elite athletic activity.[6] In a study of midfoot sprains in collegiate football players, this injury was found to be the second most-common foot injury, occurring in 4% of players annually. Twenty-nine percent of these injuries occurred in offensive linemen.[7] Faciszewski and colleagues[6] studied subtle injuries of the Lisfranc joint and found that 60% of patients sustained low-energy trauma (twisting mechanism), with greater than half of these injuries being sports related. Despite being associated with relatively minor radiographic changes, subtle injury can be a source of considerable morbidity in athletes. In one series, three of nineteen patients were unable to return to their sport, and one patient went on to require fusion of the TMT joint.[8] Up to 20% of Lisfranc injuries can be overlooked or misdiagnosed based on initial radiographs because of a subtle diastasis. In a case series of 15 athletes who had Lisfranc injuries, 50% (4 out of 8) of the patients that had initial non-weight-bearing radiographs that appeared normal later demonstrated diastasis seen on weight-bearing radiographs.[5] An understanding of the anatomy, clinical presentation, and mechanism of injury is necessary to provide appropriate treatment for these injuries.

---

[a] The Orthopaedic Center, 927 Franklin Street, Huntsville, AL 35801, USA
[b] Duke University Medical Center, Box 3000, Durham, NC 27710, USA
[c] IRCCS Galeazzi, Divisione di Chirurgia del Piede e della Caviglia, Milano, Italy
[d] Duke Health Center, 3116 North Duke Street, Room 243, Durham, NC 27704, USA
* Corresponding author.
E-mail address: easle004@mc.duke.edu (M. Easley).

Foot Ankle Clin N Am 14 (2009) 169–186
doi:10.1016/j.fcl.2009.03.008
1083-7515/09/$ – see front matter © 2009 Elsevier Inc. All rights reserved.

EPIDEMIOLOGY
General Trauma

Lisfranc joint injuries are relatively uncommon, accounting for 0.2% of all fractures, with a reported incidence rate of 1 per 55,000 people in the United States annually.[9,10] They are typically the result of a high-energy trauma, such as motor vehicle accidents and falls from heights, and 58% of them are associated with polytrauma. In a review of 76 cases of Lisfranc fractures and dislocations, two thirds were due to motor vehicle collision, with crush injury and fall from a height accounting for the next-largest number of incidences.[4] Vuori and colleagues[11] reported on Lisfranc injuries related to low-energy injuries in 32% of patients, compared with 33% due to high-energy motor vehicle collisions. Almost 40% of Lisfranc fracture dislocations in patients who had polytrauma are not recognized, and 20% are misdiagnosed.[12] This may contribute to the gross underestimation of these injuries, which are most common in the third decade of life, with males being affected two to four times more often than females.

Sport

Midfoot sprains are one of the most common athletic foot injuries, second only to injury to the metatarsophalangeal joint.[13] Direct injury occurs when a crushing load is applied directly to the midfoot. More often, injury is caused indirectly through an axial longitudinal force applied to the foot in a plantar-flexed and slightly rotated position, followed by a forceful abduction, or twisting movement.[14] This is the most common mechanism for Lisfranc sports injuries and has been reported in people involved in soccer, football, gymnastics, horseback riding, windsurfing, basketball, baseball, ballet, and running. Patients often recall an acute traumatic episode associated with a twisting injury to the foot in an awkward position. Ecchymosis extending into the toes and diffuse midfoot swelling may be present. Traumatic dislocation may occur secondary to failure of the weaker dorsal and interosseous ligaments at the TMT joints. People engaged in noncontact sports are also subject to this injury. Women's gymnastics has been one of the highest injury-producing sports and ranks first among injuries sustained that require surgery.[15] In addition, the ankle and foot are first and third, respectively, in body regions injured in women's gymnastics. In a series of 14 foot and ankle injuries, five Lisfranc injuries were reported, three that were the result of a fall from the balance beam and two from the vault. The injuries sustained on the beam were due to a direct, traumatic blow from the beam itself. Of these gymnasts, only one was able to return to the sport. In equestrian sports, injuries are the result of forced abduction caused by either falling from the horse with the foot trapped in the stirrup or by having the foot caught between the animal and ground.[16]

Unlike football and gymnastics, Lisfranc injuries are rare in dancers. This may be explained by a combination of internal and external stabilizing forces. In the full-pointe position, the TMT joints are perpendicular to the longitudinal axis of weight bearing, producing more of a compressive force and less of a shear force at these joints. In a dance-related biomechanical study, it was suggested that the stability of the pointe shoe, combined with a high level of training and muscular control in the dancer, provides a protective effect for this type of injury.[17] After sectioning the plantar ligaments in a cadaveric model, a significant improvement in stability during en-pointe loading between the middle cuneiform and the base of the second metatarsal was noted in a comparison of the shod foot and the unshod foot.

Associated Injuries

In addition to classic Lisfranc injuries at the TMT joints, there are other associated injuries or variations of injury. More frequently seen in ballerinas is a unique stress fracture of the base of the second metatarsal, which is rare in male dancers and other athletes. This suggests that significant force occurs at the base of the second metatarsal during dance that may result in stress fracture. Also, severe abduction forces causing displacement through the Lisfranc joint may result in a "nutcracker" fracture of the cuboid. With TMT dislocation, the cuboid may be crushed between the anterior calcaneus and the base of the fourth and fifth metatarsals. This type of injury can be seen in high-energy motor vehicle accidents, but it has also been reported twice in the medical literature as a relatively frequent pattern in the equestrian pediatric population.[18,19] The provision of appropriate boots or shoes with smooth soles should be made mandatory in horse riding.[20]

ANATOMY
Skeleton Description

The five metatarsal bones contribute to the long plantar arch in the sagittal plane. The TMT articulations transition more proximally in the transverse plane from medial to lateral. In the coronal plane, the base of the second metatarsal is recessed between the medial and lateral cuneiforms to create the classic "keystone" in the shape of a Roman arch, which provides inherent osseous stability. In an imaging study (level III evidence), the mortise of the Lisfranc joint between the medial and lateral cuneiform bones on an anteroposterior radiograph was analyzed. In injured patients, the articulation was significantly less deep when compared with control subjects. It was concluded that the conformation of the bony skeleton provides primary stability, whereas the strong ligamentous and musculotendinous structures provide indirect stability.[21]

Ligament Description

The base of the second metatarsal is connected to the each of the cuneiforms by the dorsal ligaments. The plantar and dorsal ligaments are oriented in three different directions: longitudinal, oblique, and transverse. The longitudinal and oblique fibers connect the tarsal bones to the proximal metatarsals. The transverse fibers connect the bases of the metatarsals proximally. Generally, the plantar ligaments are stronger than the dorsal ligaments, which may account for the dorsal direction of dislocations. In addition to the dorsal ligaments, there are two additional ligaments that extend from the medial cuneiform to the second metatarsal base in the coronal plane. There are no interosseous ligaments between the medial and middle cuneiforms. The metatarsal interosseous ligaments are some of the strongest of the ligamentous attachments associated with the Lisfranc joint; however, they are uniquely absent between the bases of the first and second metatarsals. The Lisfranc ligament is located between the medial cuneiform and the base of the second metatarsal. This is the largest of the interosseus ligaments and measures 1 cm in height by 0.5 cm in width.[22,23] Anatomic studies have demonstrated that it is also the strongest of the interosseous ligaments. In a biomechanical study, the Lisfranc ligament was found to be three times stronger than the dorsal ligaments, providing the most stability, followed by the plantar and dorsal ligaments, respectively.[24]

Columnar Theory

The midfoot can be divided into three columns. The lateral column is the most mobile and consists of the articulation between the fourth and fifth metatarsals and the cuboid. Posttraumatic instability is generally well tolerated in this column, and symptomatic arthritis is rare. The medial column consists of the navicular, the medial cuneiform, and the first metatarsal. The middle column is the most rigid, consisting of the second and third metatarsals and their respective TMT articulations.[4]

The rigidity of the medial and middle columns is essential for the foot to function effectively as a lever arm during normal gait. The Lisfranc ligament links the medial cuneiform to the second metatarsal, rigidly connecting the medial and middle columns while still allowing mobility between the first two metatarsals.[25]

Range of Motion

The medial, or first column, axis of motion passes through the foot in anterior, lateral, and plantar orientations. It has an inclination of 45° in the frontal and sagittal planes; however, the angle with the coronal plane is not significant, and coronal motion is limited. In the frontal and sagittal planes, there is from 3° to 4° of movement, and dorsiflexion is linked with inversion, whereas plantar flexion is associated with eversion. The lateral column demonstrates increased mobility, with up to 10° of motion in the frontal and sagittal planes. The middle column is the least mobile, given that this region is under the highest forces during the heel-rise phase of the gait.[26]

Adjacent Anatomy

The perforating branch of the dorsalis pedis traverses toward the plantar area as it passes between the bases of the first and second metatarsals. The deep peroneal nerve follows a similar course and provides sensation to the first dorsal web space. The anterior tibial tendon courses along the medial column and has a broad insertion on the dorsomedial aspect of the base of the first metatarsal and the medial cuneiform. Entrapment of the tibialis anterior tendon has been reported as preventing a closed reduction of the Lisfranc joint.[27]

CLASSIFICATIONS
Myerson Classification

Historically, the most common classification system used was described by Myerson.[4] It is an evolution of the classifications proposed by Hardcastle[3] and by Quenu and Kuss.[28] Type A injuries represent total incongruity of the TMT joint with all metatarsals displaced in the same plane or direction. In type B1, first ray displacement occurs in relative isolation, in contrast to type B2, in which displacement affects one or more of the lateral four metatarsals in any plane. In type C1, which involves a divergent pattern, the first metatarsal is displaced medially, and the lateral four metatarsals can be in any other concomitant pattern of displacement, seen with partial incongruity. Type C2 represents a divergent pattern with total incongruity. The advantage to this system is a high degree of interobserver reliability to communicate data. This classification does not provide treatment direction or outcome stratification on the basis of fracture patterns and cannot be used to reliably predict clinical results.[25,29,30]

Nunley and Vertullo[5] proposed a classification system that addresses the more-subtle, low-energy injures seen in athletics. Lisfranc sport injuries classically affect the ligamentous structures and may be associated with small fleck or avulsion fractures. They are primarily soft tissue injuries, and although there is no fracture, injured individuals can suffer tremendous pain and an inability to bear weight on the affected extremity. This classification system guides treatment of the low-energy Lisfranc sprains based on clinical findings, comparative weight-bearing radiographs, and bone scans (**Fig. 1**).

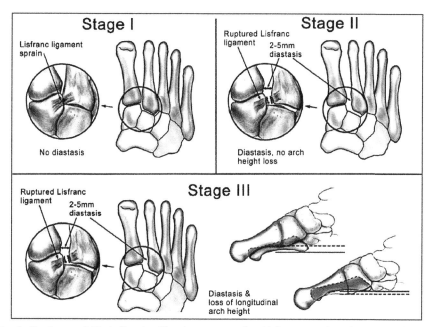

Fig. 1. Nunley and Vertullo classification system for Lisfranc sprains. (*From* Nunley JA, Vertullo CJ. Classification, investigation, and management of midfoot sprains: Lisfranc injuries in the athlete. Am J Sports Med 2002;30:871; with permission.)

Stage I is a sprain of the Lisfranc ligament with no measurable diastasis between the medial cuneiform and the base of the second metatarsal or loss of arch height on weight-bearing radiographs. Bone scintigrams will show increased uptake. This injury represents a dorsal capsular tear and sprain without elongation of the Lisfranc ligament. The Lisfranc complex is stable. stage II sprains result in diastasis of 1 mm to 5 mm between the base of the second metatarsal and the medial cuneiform. The dorsal ligament and interosseous ligaments are injured; however, there is no loss of arch height. Elongation or disruption of the Lisfranc ligament can be present, but the plantar capsular structures remain intact (**Fig. 2**). Stage III sprains result in diastasis of greater than 5mm and loss of arch height. This is represented by a decreased or negative value of the distance between the plantar aspect of the fifth metatarsal bone and the plantar aspect of the medial cuneiform bone on a weight-bearing lateral radiograph.[6] This injury may be associated with more-significant displacement, and in such cases, the Myerson classification should be used to describe the injury.

IMAGING
Standard Radiographs

Initial imaging should consist of anteroposterior, 30° oblique, and lateral radiographs of the affected foot. Weight-bearing views should be obtained to provide stress across the injury to check for diastasis caused by ligamentous injury. When weight bearing is limited by pain, ankle block anesthesia can be used.[5,6] There is no study that defines how much weight is necessary to define a radiograph as a weight-bearing study.[31] Comparison views can also be helpful, provided the contralateral foot is uninjured. Radiographs should also be examined for associated fractures, which occur in 39% of patients who have Lisfranc injuries.[11]

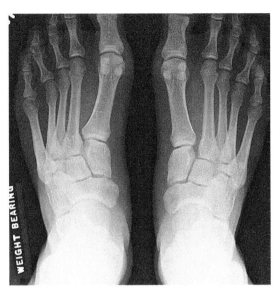

Fig. 2. Comparison anteroposterior weight-bearing radiograph demonstrating diastasis between the base of the second metatarsal and the medial cuneiform on the right foot.

In an uninjured foot, the medial aspect of the base of the second metatarsal should be aligned with the medial aspect of the medial cuneiform on the anteroposterior view. The medial aspect of the fourth metatarsal base should be aligned with the medial aspect of the cuboid on the oblique view. On the lateral view, the dorsal surface of the first and second metatarsals should be level with the corresponding cuneiforms. The most consistent radiographic finding in Lisfranc joint injuries is the loss of alignment of the medial border of the second metatarsal with the medial border of the middle cuneiform.[32] Four additional observation points include (1) the distance between the first and second metatarsal bones, (2) the distance between the medial and intermediate cuneiform bones on an anteroposterior radiograph, (3) the distance between the plantar aspect of the fifth metatarsal and the plantar medial cuneiform bones on a lateral radiograph, and (4) the presence of avulsion fractures (fleck sign).[5] Comparisons should be made with the contralateral foot, and any diastasis that is 1 mm greater than that of structures in the uninjured foot should be considered diagnostic.

Additional Imaging

Bone scans are useful for stage 1 injuries[5] and can show minor metabolic and blood flow changes when other imaging modalities demonstrate normal results. Additionally, they may show increase uptake in the region of injury for up to 1 year after the injury or event.

Some authors suggest the use of CT and MRI, however these imaging studies are generally not weight bearing, and in nondisplaced injuries, may provide little additional benefit. CT scans are useful to assess fracture comminution and are more commonly used in high-energy Lisfranc joint injures.[33,34] The usefulness of the MRI will depend on the expertise of the physician who is interpreting the films. Raikin and colleagues, compared MRI findings to intraoperative stress radiographs and surgical findings and determined that magnetic resonance imaging is accurate for detecting traumatic injury of the Lisfranc ligament. It is useful to assess Lisfranc joint complex instability when the plantar Lisfranc ligament bundle is used as a predictor. The appearance of a normal ligament is suggestive of a stable midfoot, and documentation of its integrity may obviate the need for a manual stress radiographic evaluation under anesthesia for a patient with equivocal clinical and radiographic examinations.[35]

Stress Radiographs

Many authors advocate using stress radiographs for both acute and nonacute injuries. Abduction stress radiographs allow the examiner to dynamically visualize the space between the second metatarsal and second cuneiform and the space between the first cuneiform and the second metatarsal and cuneiform (longitudinal). This represents dorsal displacement and might allow visualization of abnormal movement that could lead to posttraumatic arthritis. Subtle first cuneiform–second metatarsal diastasis is difficult to detect using abduction stress radiographs because the direction of the x-ray beam is often too oblique with respect to the joints of interest, resulting in difficulty determining the actual diastasis.[36] The failure to detect a first cuneiform–second metatarsal diastasis may also be the result of dorsal translation of the first cuneiform, which may cause the three-dimensional diastasis to appear more vertically oriented.

CONSERVATIVE TREATMENT

Lisfranc joint sprains and fractures should be referred to surgeons who have specific interest either in trauma or in foot and ankle surgery. Nunley and Vertullo stage I sprains can be treated using a non–weight-bearing cast for 6 weeks, followed by the use of custom-molded orthotics. This treatment may be successful for patients who have been misdiagnosed for up to 8 months. If pain continues after cast removal, consider using a removable boot for 4 additional weeks.[5]

Some authors suggest conservative treatment for all painful injuries that do not show displacement on stress views. Stress views should be repeated 10 to 14 days after the initial injury. If stability is maintained, treatment should continue for 6 weeks of immobilization in a short leg cast, with the foot in a relaxed, slightly inverted position. Conversion to a removable fracture boot may be possible after 6 weeks, with progressive weight bearing as tolerated.[37]

For isolated ligamentous disruptions, the duration of immobilization may need to be 3 to 4 months to prevent displacement. Range-of-motion exercises can be initiated at 6 to 8 weeks. Progressive weight bearing can begin at 3 months, with physical therapy as needed. A molded, cushioned insert with cushioned, supportive running footwear should be used. Communication with the patient plays a central role in the treatment of these injuries. The patient should have a clear understanding that the injury is not a common ankle sprain and that in elite athletes it may result in a prolonged course of recovery after injury.[25]

SURGICAL TREATMENT
Indications

Nunley and Vertullo stage II injuries should be treated operatively with an initial attempt of closed reduction under fluoroscopy. Screw fixation is preferred, using either partially threaded, cannulated 3.5-mm or 4.5-mm screws (dependent on patient size) or fully threaded, noncannulated screws. In a review of 19 athletes, open reduction and internal fixation was preferred for all patients who had diastasis, regardless of degree, despite the risk of arthritis that may be sustained from an intra-articular screw.[8] Stiffness is preferred in lieu of instability to provide a rigid lever to the medial column during gait and activity.

Myerson type B1 injuries should be fixed using a screw inserted from the medial cuneiform into the base of the second metatarsal and from the medial cuneiform into the intermediate cuneiform bone. Type B2 injuries should be fixed using a percutaneous screw from the medial cuneiform into the base of the second metatarsal bone.

Open Reduction Internal Fixation Compared with Arthrodesis

The most important goal of surgery for Lisfranc injuries should be the anatomic reduction of the TMT joints. Arthrodesis has been reserved as a salvage procedure after the failure of open reduction and internal fixation, after a delayed or missed diagnosis, or for severely comminuted intra-articular fractures of the TMT joints with a high suspicion of risk for posttraumatic arthritis.

Some authors advocate arthrodesis as the treatment of choice for Lisfranc complex injuries. In one study of 41 patients with primarily ligamentous injury, patients treated using open reduction internal fixation (ORIF) tended to have greater loss of correction, greater deformity, and more degenerative changes than those treated using primary arthrodesis. However, arthrodesis was contraindicated for subtle injuries with minimal or no displacement.[38] Kuo and colleagues[39] also suggested that some patients with purely ligamentous Lisfranc injuries may be better treated using primary fusion. Mulier and colleagues[40] advocated the use of open reduction and internal fixation or partial arthrodesis for severe Lisfranc injuries, and they stated that primary complete arthrodesis should be reserved for cases of severely comminuted fractures or as a salvage procedure.

Lateral Column Treatment

The literature is in agreement on the treatment of the lateral column. When the fourth and fifth TMTs are well reduced, no procedure is necessary; however, when they are not well reduced, percutaneous reduction using Kirschner-wires (K-wires) should be performed, with removal after 6 weeks. The goal is to preserve motion in the lateral column to allow normal gait and to avoid overloading of the lateral column as the result of an iatrogenic stiff foot. Posttraumatic arthritis is rarely symptomatic in these joints.

SURGICAL TECHNIQUE

Regardless of the choice of using osteosynthesis or arthrodesis, the goal is to obtain an anatomic reduction. Fixation is described in three variations. The second metatarsal base is used as a keystone in the first variation. The joint is reduced and held in place using a large, Weber, pointed reduction clamp. The base of the second metatarsal is lagged through the medial cuneiform in line with the normal Lisfranc ligament. After stabilization, if the first metatarsophalangeal joint is unstable, it is fixed using another screw, placed distal to proximal, using either a fully threaded or partially threaded positioning screw. It is important to countersink this screw head to prevent dorsal fracture of the base of the first metatarsal. The third metatarsal is secured to the middle or lateral cuneiform from distal to proximal. Alternatively, each joint is anatomically reduced and provisional fixation is accomplished using wires. Stabilization of each metatarsal to its proximal articulation is then achieved using non-lag screw fixation. A third alternative is commonly used in Europe. In this option, any plantar fragments in the base of the second metatarsal are reduced and lagged from the dorsal aspect of the metatarsal. The TMT joints are then reduced, and non-lag screws are placed across each of the TMT joints, including the fourth and fifth. The screws are left in place for only 8 weeks, after which all the screws are removed. There is a concern that this technique leads to a higher incidence of late displacement because of the early removal of the screws.[37]

TIMING

The soft tissue envelope is respected, and surgical timing is delayed until the skin wrinkles, indicating that the swelling has subsided. Compartment syndrome is less likely in sports injuries than crush injuries. However, if it is present, fasciotomy is indicated for injuries of the foot.[25] Prompt diagnosis and treatment may allow for improved outcome and better healing potential.

SURGICAL APPROACH
Longitudinal Incision

Sangeorzan and Hansen describe the use of two incisions: a straight or lazy-S incision over the second TMT joint and a second incision between the third and fourth TMT joints, with the addition of a third, more-lateral incision when the lateral column is involved.[41] Alternatively, a more medial incision is made that is deepened through the anterior tibial tendon retinaculum and subsequently repaired at the end of the procedure. The incision may also be extended if an extensive arthrodesis that includes the navicular–cuneiform joint is addressed. The extensor hallucis brevis tendon lies directly over the neurovascular bundle, which is retracted medially. A more-lateral second incision, which is centered over the midfoot, may be used in cases of involvement of the third TMT joint. In cases of lateral column involvement, a third incision, using the interval between the sural and superficial peroneal nerve, allows exposure of the fourth and fifth TMT articulations with the cuboid.

In a meta-analysis, Desmond and Chou[25] recommended a medial or dorsal incision over the first TMT joint while avoiding the first intermetatarsal space to protect the dorsalis pedis artery and deep peroneal nerve. The second incision is positioned between the second and third TMT joints, and a third incision may be added between the fourth and fifth TMT joints when the lateral column is involved. Arntz and colleagues[42] suggested placing the medial incision in the first web space, but taking care to create full-thickness skin flaps to protect the dorsalis pedis artery under the skin bridge to prevent necrosis of the skin bridge, and they proposed placing the lateral incision between the fourth and fifth metatarsals. As an alternative, they suggested the Hannover approach, in which the incision is extended from the second web space proximally to the extensor retinaculum. The incision may then be extended proximally towards the knee when necessary.

Transverse Incision

Mann and colleagues[43] noted that wound necrosis and limited access to the TMT joints are two common problems encountered in the approach to the Lisfranc joint. A novel transverse incision has been described as a solution to these problems. The transverse incision lies in a zone of the midfoot that is proximal to the arcuate artery and distal to the lateral tarsal artery. It preserves the dorsalis pedis artery, minimizing the disruption to the midfoot's cutaneous blood supply. Surgical exposure is performed using six different intervals to gain exposure to the Lisfranc joint. The exposure is ideal when the injury is more severe and involves multiple TMT joints. In a series of 12 patients, wound complications were not seen in patients for whom various forms of immunosuppression were used.[44]

ARTHROSCOPIC APPROACH

Although uncommon, arthroscopic reduction using five portals has been described. The first is a portal medial to the first TMT joint that allows access to the plantar medial aspect of the first TMT joint. The remaining portals are interosseous and include P1–2 (the junction point between the medial cuneiform and the first and second metatarsals) to explore the second TMT joint; P2–3 (the junction point between the second metatarsal and the intermediate and lateral cuneiforms) for the third TMT joint; P3–4 (the junction point between the cuboid, the lateral cuneiform, and the third and fourth metatarsals) for the fourth and fifth TMTs; and P4–5 (the junction point between the proximal articular surfaces of the fourth and fifth metatarsals).[45]

AUTHORS' PREFERRED APPROACH

In the approach preferred by the authors of this article, the patient is placed supine on the operating room table with a calf tourniquet. An attempt at closed reduction under fluoroscopic guidance is performed. A large, pointed reduction clamp is used for the reduction, with the points positioned at the lateral aspect of the base of the second metatarsal and the medial aspect of the medial cuneiform (**Fig. 3**). If the joint is anatomically reduced, a fully threaded, percutaneous 3.5-mm screw is placed from the medial cuneiform to the base of the second metatarsal. If the joint cannot be anatomically reduced using percutaneous attempts, then an open approach is used. The joint is exposed through the interval between the extensor hallucis longus tendon and the deep neurovascular bundle. The dorsal interosseous ligaments will be visibly torn (**Fig. 4**). A rongeur can be used to remove tissue that prohibits anatomic reduction (**Fig. 5**). If necessary, K-wires are used to assist with provisional fixation (**Fig. 6**). When the joint is anatomically reduced, a guide wire is placed from the medial cuneiform to the base of the second metatarsal and a cannulated drill is used to drill the medial cuneiform only (**Fig. 7**). Before drilling, a guide pin is advanced through the skin on the dorsum of the foot to prevent the possibility of difficulty in removing a broken guide pin associated with drilling. After the medial cuneiform has been drilled, the guide pin is removed and a 2.5-mm drill bit is used to drill into the base of the second metatarsal. The appropriate-length screw is selected and then advanced from the medial cuneiform to the base of the second metatarsal. Care is

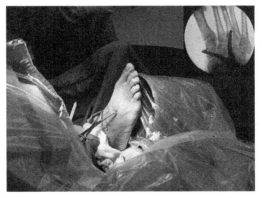

Fig. 3. In the authors' preferred technique for percutaneous reduction, a large, pointed reduction clamp is used.

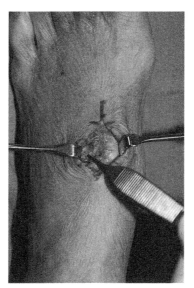

Fig. 4. Torn dorsal Lisfranc ligaments.

taken to protect the soft tissues to avoid interposition of the tibialis anterior between the bone and screw (**Fig. 8**). Stability is examined in adjacent joints, and if there is instability between the cuneiforms or at the first TMT joints, these joints are stabilized using screw fixation. **Fig. 9** is an anteroposterior radiograph that demonstrates complete reduction of the diastasis in a collegiate lacrosse player.

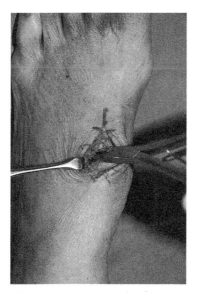

Fig. 5. A rongeur can be used to remove interposed soft tissue.

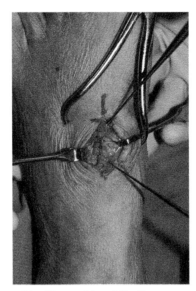

Fig. 6. K-wires are used to assist with provisional fixation.

FIXATION CHOICE
Screws

Internal fixation has been described using cortical 4.5-mm and 3.5-mm screws with or without lag technique. Some authors support the use of 3.5-mm screws with no lag technique because it presents less risk of arthritis.[39,40] Screws across the third TMT joint fail most often. This is most likely caused by the close proximity of the third TMT joint to the more-mobile fourth and fifth TMT joints. Screws across the first TMT joint had the second-highest prevalence of failure. The addition of a second screw from proximal to distal added rotational stability, prevented plantar gapping, and decreased the rate of screw breakage.[41]

Plates

Plate fixation may minimize intraoperative trauma to the articular surfaces of the TMT joint and theoretically help to improve patient outcome by allowing earlier

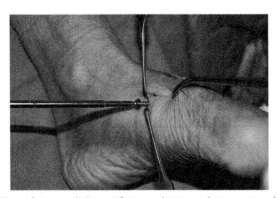

Fig. 7. During drilling of the medial cuneiform and screw advancement, the soft tissues are protected to avoid entrapment of the tibialis anterior tendon.

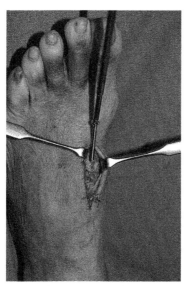

Fig. 8. Tissues are protected to avoid entrapment of the tibialis anterior tendon.

postoperative range of motion. In a study comparing the use of plantar plating to the use of transarticular screws, it was found that plantar plating was stiffer and sustained less displacement from initial to final loading.[46] A biomechanical study demonstrated that dorsal plating resulted in a less stable construct compared with plantar plating, and was comparable to the use of transarticular screws.[47] The primary concern with dorsal plating is soft tissue irritation postoperatively. Newer plate designs with low-profile plates and screw heads have decreased soft tissue irritation.

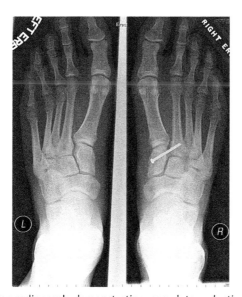

Fig. 9. Anteroposterior radiograph demonstrating complete reduction of the diastasis in a collegiate lacrosse player.

Kirschner Wires

K-wires should be used frequently for provisional fixation or temporarily in cases of severe comminution in which screw purchase is poor. This is the preferred fixation method used for the lateral column to allow for anatomic healing without compromising mobility of the fourth and fifth TMT articulations.

New Materials

Bioabsorbable materials, such as polylactide screws, avoid the need for subsequent surgery to remove hardware. In a clinical study, the use of absorbable screws was found to be safe and without reaction, and their use obviated the need for screw removal at short-term follow-up.[48] Biomechanical studies have demonstrated acceptable stiffness in other anatomic regions, such as the tibiofibular syndesomosis, when they were fixed using bioabsorbable screws.[49]

COMPLICATIONS

The most common problem resulting from Lisfranc injury is posttraumatic arthritis. Failure to diagnosis the injury or malreduction increases the risk of posttraumatic arthritis. Kuo and colleagues[39] (level IV evidence) observed a 25% rate of arthritis in their series, and 50% (6/12) of those patients were treated using arthrodesis. Myerson and collagues,[4] in their largest Lisfranc series (level IV evidence), reported an additional 27 operations on 20 patients at an average of 18 months: 17 of the 27 procedures were performed using arthrodesis. Other procedures that were performed included exostectomy, neuroma resection, tendon lengthening, and skin grafting. Sangeorzan and colleagues[50] treated 16 patients who failed initial treatment using salvage arthrodesis. The deformity was reduced, and lag screw fixation was used to stabilize the arthrodesis. Good to excellent results were achieved in 11 patients, and fair or poor results in 5 (level IV evidence). Although it is important to treat symptomatic arthritic joints, preservation of lateral column mobility achieved by avoidance of fourth and fifth TMT arthrodesis is advised.

Additional complications described included complex regional pain syndrome, symptomatic hardware, injuries to the superficial or deep peroneal nerve manifested as a sensory deficit, hardware failure, incomplete or loss of reduction, deep venous thrombosis, infection, nonunion, and malunion.[29]

POSTOPERATIVE TREATMENT

In general, the extremity is placed in a well-padded dressing with a plaster posterior splint or a removable boot until suture removal at 2 weeks. The patient remains non-weight bearing in a short leg cast or boot for an additional 4 to 10 weeks, depending on the injury. For a subtle Lisfranc injury in an athlete, weight bearing may be initiated at 6 weeks using a removable boot and accommodative orthotic. Temporary K-wires are typically removed at 6 weeks and should be removed before weight bearing to prevent pin breakage. Different authors suggest that screw removal may be scheduled from 6 months to 12 months following surgery.[5]

OUTCOMES

In the literature, there are no significant differences with respect to outcome for age, gender, and cause of injury. Anatomic reduction and early treatment significantly affect the outcome.[7] Current available level IV evidence demonstrates an American Orthopaedic Foot and Ankle Society score between 68 and 72. Myerson and colleagues[4] (in their largest series of 76 patients) and Arntz and colleagues[42] (28 good results in 30 patients, with an average follow-up of 3.4 years) found that the quality of the initial reduction is the most important factor for excellent or good clinical results.

When comparing the use of ORIF with that of arthrodesis, Richter and colleagues[51] did not find a significant difference in the method of treatment at an 8.5-year follow-up. They suggested that the restoration of the columns is very important, as reflected by the high correlation between correct column length and good functional outcome. They also suggested that treatment should be dictated by the condition of the soft tissue envelope and that repeated attempts of closed reduction should be avoided. In a case series with follow-up at an average of 30.1 months, Mulier and colleagues[40] found that ORIF demonstrated good or excellent results in 65% of cases, compared with 45% in the arthrodesis group. Nonunion was also present in 33% of cases in the complete arthrodesis group. Reflex sympathetic dystrophy, stiffness in the forefoot, and difficulty in wearing shoes were seen more frequently in patients in the complete arthrodesis group compared with those in the ORIF or partial arthrodesis groups; however, these differences were not statistically significant, and therefore it was concluded that there was no difference in outcomes between the cases using partial arthrodesis and ORIF.

Conservative treatment in athletes who have Nunley and Vertullo stage I Lisfranc injuries is supported by other reported outcomes in the literature. Meyer and colleagues[7] reported on 23 athletic sprains, of which only three demonstrated diastasis. Shapiro and colleagues[52] reported on nine athletes who had type B1 injuries; they treated only one using patient using surgery. Excellent results were reported, with athletes returning to their sport at 3 months. Conservative treatment does not offer a more rapid return to sports when compared with operative management.[5]

FUNCTIONAL EVALUATION

In Richter's series, pedobarographic measurement results correlated with patient subjective outcomes. Only patients who did not have considerable symptoms showed a normal or near normal gait pattern.[51] The results of the gait analysis, using the F-Scan in-shoe pressure monitoring system (Tekscan, Inc, Boston, Massachusetts), as performed by Teng and colleagues,[53] did not show a significant difference between the injured and the noninjured foot in 11 patients.

SUMMARY

Lisfranc complex problems represent a broad spectrum of injuries. There should be a high index of suspicion of this injury, and prompt diagnosis is important to allow athletes to return to their sport with the best possible outcome. Nonoperative treatment is reserved for stage I sprains. The goal of operative treatment is to achieve a stable anatomic reduction. In non or minimally displaced injuries, reduction may be performed percutaneously; however, if a perfect reduction cannot be obtained, formal ORIF is recommended. Primary arthrodesis should be reserved as a salvage procedure for complex injuries with intra-articular comminution or significant displacement. A gradual return to athletics with sports-specific training is important to prevent reinjury. Despite appropriate treatment, subjective outcomes may not parallel the radiographic outcomes, and patients should be aware of the severity of the injury.

REFERENCES

1. Cassebaum WH. Lisfranc fracture-dislocations. Clin Orthop Relat Res 1963;30: 116.
2. Fischer L. Jacques Lisfranc de Saint-Martin (1787–1847). Hist Sci Med 2005;39:17.
3. Hardcastle PH, Reschauer R, Kutscha-Lissberg E, et al. Injuries to the TMT joint. Incidence, classification and treatment. J Bone Joint Surg Br 1982;64:349.
4. Myerson MS, Fisher RT, Burgess AR, et al. Fracture dislocations of the TMT joints: end results correlated with pathology and treatment. Foot Ankle 1986;6:225.
5. Nunley JA, Vertullo CJ. Classification, investigation, and management of midfoot sprains: Lisfranc injuries in the athlete. Am J Sports Med 2002;30:871.
6. Faciszewski T, Burks RT, Manaster BJ. Subtle injuries of the Lisfranc joint. J Bone Joint Surg Am 1990;72:1519.
7. Meyer SA, Callaghan JJ, Albright JP, et al. Midfoot sprains in collegiate football players. Am J Sports Med 1994;22:392.
8. Curtis MJ, Myerson M, Szura B. Tarsometatarsal joint injuries in the athlete. Am J Sports Med 1993;21:497.
9. Aitken AP, Poulson D. Dislocations of the TMT joint. J Bone Joint Surg Am 1963; 45-A:246.
10. English TA. Dislocations of the metatarsal bone and adjacent toe. J Bone Joint Surg Br 1964;46:700.
11. Vuori JP, Aro HT. Lisfranc joint injuries: trauma mechanisms and associated injuries. J Trauma 1993;35:40.
12. Jarde O, Gaffuri JG, Woestelandt T, et al. [Fractures-luxations of the Lisfranc joint. Apropos of 39 cases]. Ann Radiol (Paris) 1991;34(4):278–84 [in French].
13. Clanton T. Athletic injuries to the soft tissues of the foot and ankle. 7th edition. St Louis (MO): Mosby; 1999.
14. Harwood MI, Raikin SM. A Lisfranc fracture-dislocation in a football player. J Am Board Fam Pract 2003;16:69.
15. Chilvers M, Donahue M, Nassar L, et al. Foot and ankle injuries in elite female gymnasts. Foot Ankle Int 2007;28:214.
16. Ceroni D, De Rosa V, De Coulon G, et al. The importance of proper shoe gear and safety stirrups in the prevention of equestrian foot injuries. J Foot Ankle Surg 2007;46:32.
17. Kadel N, Boenisch M, Teitz C, et al. Stability of Lisfranc joints in ballet pointe position. Foot Ankle Int 2005;26:394.
18. Hermel MB, Gershon-Cohen J. The nutcracker fracture of the cuboid by indirect violence. Radiology 1953;60:850.
19. Hsu JC, Chang JH, Wang SJ, et al. The nutcracker fracture of the cuboid in children: a case report. Foot Ankle Int 2004;25:423.
20. Bentley T, Page S, Meyer D, et al. How safe is adventure tourism in New Zealand? An exploratory analysis. Appl Ergon 2001;32:327.
21. Peicha G, Labovitz J, Seibert FJ, et al. The anatomy of the joint as a risk factor for Lisfranc dislocation and fracture-dislocation. An anatomical and radiological case control study. J Bone Joint Surg Br 2002;84:981.
22. de Palma L, Santucci A, Sabetta SP, et al. Anatomy of the Lisfranc joint complex. Foot Ankle Int 1997;18:356.
23. Milankov M, Miljkovic N, Popovic N. Concomitant plantar TMT (Lisfranc) and metatarsophalangeal joint dislocations. Arch Orthop Trauma Surg 2003;123:95.
24. Solan MC, Moorman CT III, Miyamoto RG, et al. Ligamentous restraints of the second TMT joint: a biomechanical evaluation. Foot Ankle Int 2001;22:637.

25. Desmond EA, Chou LB. Current concepts review: Lisfranc injuries. Foot Ankle Int 2006;27:653.
26. Root MI. Biomechanical examination of the foot. J Am Podiatry Assoc 1973;63:28.
27. DeBenedetti MJ, Evanski PM, Waugh TR. The unreducible Lisfranc fracture. Case report and literature review. Clin Orthop Relat Res 1978;136:238–40.
28. Quenu E, Kuss G. Etude sur les luxations du metatose. Rev Chir 1909;39: 231–336.
29. Komenda GA, Myerson MS, Biddinger KR. Results of arthrodesis of the TMT joints after traumatic injury. J Bone Joint Surg Am 1996;78:1665.
30. Talarico RH, Hamilton GA, Ford LA, et al. Fracture dislocations of the TMT joints: analysis of interrater reliability in using the modified Hardcastle classification system. J Foot Ankle Surg 2006;45:300.
31. Mullen JE, O'Malley MJ. Sprains—residual instability of subtalar, Lisfranc joints, and turf toe. Clin Sports Med 2004;23:97.
32. Foster SC, Foster RR. Lisfranc's TMT fracture-dislocation. Radiology 1976;120: 79.
33. Haapamaki V, Kiuru M, Koskinen S. Lisfranc fracture-dislocation in patients with multiple trauma: diagnosis with multidetector computed tomography. Foot Ankle Int 2004;25:614.
34. Potter HG, Deland JT, Gusmer PB, et al. Magnetic resonance imaging of the Lisfranc ligament of the foot. Foot Ankle Int 1998;19:438.
35. Raikin SM, Elias I, Dheer S, et al. Prediction of midfoot instability in the subtle Lisfranc injury: Comparison of magnetic resonance imaging with intraoperative findings. J Bone Joint Surg Am 2009;91:892–9.
36. Coss HS, Manos RE, Buoncristiani A, et al. Abduction stress and AP weightbearing radiography of purely ligamentous injury in the TMT joint. Foot Ankle Int 1998; 19:537.
37. Sands AK, Grose A. Lisfranc injuries. Injury 2004;35(Suppl 2):SB71.
38. Ly TV, Coetzee JC. Treatment of primarily ligamentous Lisfranc joint injuries: primary arthrodesis compared with open reduction and internal fixation. A prospective, randomized study. J Bone Joint Surg Am 2006;88:514.
39. Kuo RS, Tejwani NC, Digiovanni CW, et al. Outcome after open reduction and internal fixation of Lisfranc joint injuries. J Bone Joint Surg Am 2000;82-A: 1609.
40. Mulier T, Reynders P, Sioen W, et al. The treatment of Lisfranc injuries. Acta Orthop Belg 1997;63:82.
41. Sangeorzan BJ, Hansen ST. Cuneiform-metatarsal (Lisfranc) arthrodesis. 2nd edition. Philadelphia: Lippincott Williams & Wilkins; 2002. p. 237–52.
42. Arntz CT, Veith RG, Hansen ST Jr. Fractures and fracture-dislocations of the TMT joint. J Bone Joint Surg Am 1988;70:173.
43. Mann RA, Prieskorn D, Sobel M. Mid-tarsal and TMT arthrodesis for primary degenerative osteoarthrosis or osteoarthrosis after trauma. J Bone Joint Surg Am 1996;78:1376.
44. Vertullo CJ, Easley ME, Nunley JA. The transverse dorsal approach to the Lisfranc joint. Foot Ankle Int 2002;23:420.
45. Lui TH. Arthroscopic TMT (Lisfranc) arthrodesis. Knee Surg Sports Traumatol Arthrosc 2007;15:671.
46. Marks RM, Parks BG, Schon LC. Midfoot fusion technique for neuroarthropathic feet: biomechanical analysis and rationale. Foot Ankle Int 1998;19:507.
47. Sangeorzan BJ, Hansen ST Jr. Early and late posttraumatic foot reconstruction. Clin Orthop Relat Res 1989;243:86–91.

48. Thordarson DB, Hurvitz G. PLA screw fixation of Lisfranc injuries. Foot Ankle Int 2002;23:1003.
49. Thordarson DB, Hedman TP, Gross D, et al. Biomechanical evaluation of polylactide absorbable screws used for syndesmosis injury repair. Foot Ankle Int 1997; 18:622.
50. Sangeorzan BJ, Veith RG, Hansen ST Jr. Salvage of Lisfranc's TMT joint by arthrodesis. Foot Ankle 1990;10:193.
51. Richter M, Wippermann B, Krettek C, et al. Fractures and fracture dislocations of the midfoot: occurrence, causes and long-term results. Foot Ankle Int 2001;22: 392.
52. Shapiro MS, Wascher DC, Finerman GA. Rupture of Lisfranc's ligament in athletes. Am J Sports Med 1994;22:687.
53. Teng AL, Pinzur MS, Lomasney L, et al. Functional outcome following anatomic restoration of tarsal-metatarsal fracture dislocation. Foot Ankle Int 2002;23:922.

Evaluation and Treatment of Navicular Stress Fractures, Including Nonunions, Revision Surgery, and Persistent Pain After Treatment

Jeffrey A. Mann, MD[a],*, David I. Pedowitz, MS, MD[b]

KEYWORDS

- Navicular • Stress fracture • Stress reaction
- Nonunion • Arthritis

The topic of stress fractures of the tarsal navicular continues to receive attention because of its implications for high-performance professional athletes. However, the injury itself is rather uncommon. Navicular stress fractures were originally described anecdotally in 1958 in the outer front and rear legs of racing dogs, and were thought to occur because of increased stresses on the outer limbs.[1] Reports in human beings were not published for another 12 years, when in 1970 Towne and colleagues[2] presented two cases. Published reports estimate that they comprise 14% to 25% of all stress fractures, but with increasing attention to this injury and its diagnosis, these numbers may increase.[3–6] Despite increased awareness of the injury and a heightened index of suspicion by those physicians evaluating sports-related foot pain, the entity remains difficult to diagnose. The most effective treatment strategies vary considerably, depending on the patient's activity level and expectation for a return to that level.

ANATOMY, PHYSIOLOGY, BIOMECHANICS

The navicular bone is uniquely situated in the midfoot, such that it plays an integral part in a variety of joints, undergoes numerous forces, and possesses an unusual vascular supply, all of which render it susceptible to overuse injury.

[a] Department of Orthopedic Surgery, Summit Medical Center, 80 Grand Avenue, 5th floor, Oakland, CA 94612, USA
[b] Department of Orthopedic Surgery, Crystal Run Healthcare, 155 Crystal Run Road, Middletown, NY 10941, USA
* Corresponding author.
E-mail address: jeffamann@sbcglobal.net (J.A. Mann).

Foot Ankle Clin N Am 14 (2009) 187–204
doi:10.1016/j.fcl.2009.01.003
1083-7515/09/$ – see front matter © 2009 Elsevier Inc. All rights reserved.

This boat-shaped bone is convex distally and concave proximally (**Fig. 1**). It represents the base of the medial column of the foot and helps to form the proximal medial post of the transverse arch. All but its dorsal and medial surfaces are lined by articular cartilage. Proximally, it articulates with the talus; distally it articulates with the medial, middle, and lateral cuneiforms; and inferolaterally it shares an articulation with the cuboid. Its dorsal and medial surfaces serve as attachment sites for capsular, ligamentous, and tendinous structures. Specifically, the medial tuberosity provides for the major insertion of the posterior tibial tendon, while the plantar beak serves as the insertion site for the calcaneonavicular or "spring" ligament.

The navicular is susceptible to stress fractures based on specific biomechanical and vascular properties. Investigators have described a zone of maximum shear stress corresponding to the central one-third of the navicular body, where these fractures tend to occur (see **Fig. 1**).[7] It has been theorized that during the foot-strike phase of running, especially with the foot in equinus (on tiptoes), compression forces are generated from distal to proximal across the medial and lateral aspects of the navicular through the first and second metatarsocuneiform joints, respectively. The forces across the first metatarsal and medial cuneiform are directly resisted by the talar head, whereas those across the second metatarsl and middle cuneiform are not. The navicular experiences a zone of maximal shear stress between these two compression forces. This point is the central one-third of the navicular and is just lateral to the center of the talar head in the talonavicular articulation.

The blood supply to the navicular is derived dorsally from branches of the dorsalis pedis, which feed the lateral one-third, plantarly from the medial plantar artery and medially at the posterior tibial tendon insertion from contributions of both the dorsalis pedis and medial plantar artery. Combined with the aforementioned biomechanical

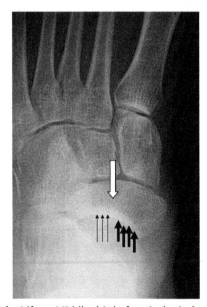

Fig.1. Plain radiograph of midfoot. Middle third of navicular is the site of shear stress (*white arrow*), because of varying resistance by the talar head and of forces transmitted through the first and second rays. The talus resists forces through the first ray (*large black arrows*), greater than forces through the second ray (*small black arrows*).

factors, because this central zone is devoid of a direct blood supply, it has difficulty healing when under repetitive stress.[8] Torg and colleagues[9] proposed that repetitive cyclical loading of the navicular in this way, combined with an as yet undetermined anatomic foot variation, results in a fatigue failure through this central area.

PATIENT PRESENTATION, HISTORY, AND PHYSICAL EXAMINATION

There is often a considerable delay in the diagnosis of navicular stress fractures because of the subtle and often vague clinical presentation of these injuries. For this reason, a mandatory high index of suspicion for navicular stress fractures should accompany the evaluation of any athlete with foot pain. Torg and colleagues[9] reported an average of 7 months between the onset of symptoms and eventual diagnosis in their series of navicular stress fractures.

As with all orthopedic complaints, evaluation of foot pain should begin with a thorough history. Clues that point one toward the diagnosis of a navicular stress fracture include the insidious onset of vague, dorsally based foot pain worse with certain activities, such as explosive sprinting, rapid changes in direction, jumping, and push-off. Sports in which these movements predominate include track and field, rugby, American football, and basketball. While errors in training are often implicated in stress-related injuries, their direct relationship with stress fractures of the navicular specifically, are unclear. Sudden increases in the intensity of activity, however, should not be overlooked, and many times do precede stress fractures.

The pain associated with navicular stress fractures is often initially only experienced during participation in a particular sport, with minimal or no symptoms with all other activities of daily living. Eventually, the discomfort evolves to include nonathletic activity and will prevent athletic participation. The discomfort typically begins as generalized pain, soreness, or cramping along the dorsum and medial midfoot. However, the patient may also present with pain localized to the ankle, forefoot, or even the plantar aspect of the foot, and may not become focally painful over the dorsal navicular itself. Initial presentation to a health care profession often results in the misdiagnosis of a midfoot sprain or tendonitis of anterior or posterior tibial tendons. In the adolescent with this history, idiopathic ischemic necrosis (Kohler's disease) should be ruled out.

Physical examination of the patient with a navicular stress fracture will often reveal focal dorsal pain over the midportion of the navicular, initially described by Khan and colleagues[5] as the "N Spot." An axial load on a plantar flexed foot, such as hopping on one leg, may reproduce the symptoms the patient encountered during athletic participation.

DIAGNOSIS AND RADIOGRAPHIC WORKUP OF NAVICULAR STRESS FRACTURES

As previously alluded to, the most important diagnostic tool for a navicular stress fracture may be a high index of suspicion. If suspected, workup should begin with a series of standing radiographs of the foot and ankle. The X-rays are carefully assessed for a visible fracture line, especially over the proximal cortex of the navicular. Other bone abnormalities should be searched for, including an accessory navicular, a talar neck bone spur, or an osteochondral defect of the talus.

Too much emphasis should not be placed on a normal appearing radiograph, however, as plain radiographs have not been found to be reliable for identifying navicular stress fractures. Khan reported normal X-rays in 67% of 128 feet in one study, and 82% of 77 feet in a second study.[5,10] Torg and colleagues and Pavlov and colleagues reported similar low rates of detection on plain x-rays.[9,11]

If a navicular stress fracture is suspected but X-rays are negative, the next step is further diagnostic workup in the form of a bone scan, CT scan, or MRI scan. There is presently no consensus as to which of these should be the next test performed.

Bone scans have been found to have a 100% sensitivity in identifying navicular stress fractures. Khan, Pavlov, Torg, and Burnes have reported positive bone scans in all of the navicular stress fractures in their series', a total of 233 patients.[5,9–12] However, despite the sensitivity of bone scans, the findings are nonspecific, and a positive finding will likely mean another test is necessary to more accurately identify the characteristics of the fracture.

CT Scans

Initially, plain tomography was used to evaluate navicular stress fractures, but their use has been completely supplanted by CT scans.[9,11] CT scans have been a remarkable tool for diagnosing navicular stress fractures, evaluating the healing of fractures, and in understanding the nature of navicular stress fractures as a whole (**Fig. 2**).

Fitch and colleagues[7] initially used tomograms for evaluating navicular stress fractures before CT scanning was widely available, and found CT superior to tomograms in evaluating the fractures. Khan and colleagues[10] evaluated all 86 patients in his series of navicular stress fractures using CT scans. Potter and colleagues[13] used CT scans to evaluate residual abnormality in the navicular following both surgical and nonsurgical treatment of 32 stress fractures.

CT scans have also been used to evaluate the healing of navicular stress fractures. Kiss and colleagues[14] studied CT scans from 55 cases of navicular stress fractures, both before and after treatment. At 6 weeks after treatment, a small subset of fractures showed dorsal cortical bridging (**Fig. 3**). By 4 months after treatment, only 32% of fractures showed firm cortical union. Twelve cases showed persistent fracture gap and were considered nonunions. A few cases showed persistent abnormalities after complete fracture healing, including medullary cysts and cortical notching (**Fig. 4**). Kiss did not correlate these healing characteristics with different treatment

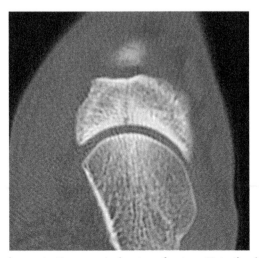

Fig. 2. Axial CT scan demonstrating a navicular stress fracture. Note the dense rim of cortical bone on the proximal cortex.

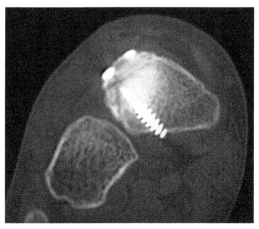

Fig. 3. CT scan image of dorsal cortical bridging after surgical repair of a navicular stress fracture.

methods, however. He concluded that CT scans were a suitable method for detecting navicular stress fractures and for following patients.

CT scans have added tremendously to the understanding of the anatomy of navicular stress fractures.[7,14] They have shown that the typical fracture is located in the central one-third of the bone, and is an incomplete fracture, not extending to the plantar cortex of the bone (**Fig. 5**). The fracture line tends to be oblique, angling from dorso-medial to plantar-lateral. Long-term follow-up has also shown that medullary cysts and cortical notching often persist after complete healing of the fracture.[14] Also characteristic is the dense, sclerotic-appearing rim of cortical bone present on the proximal articular surface of the navicular (see **Fig. 2**). This portion of the bone appears to always be involved in the stress fracture.

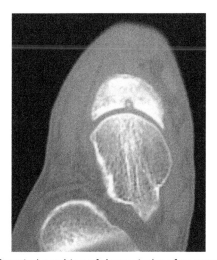

Fig. 4. CT scan image of cortical notching of the navicular after complete healing of a stress fracture.

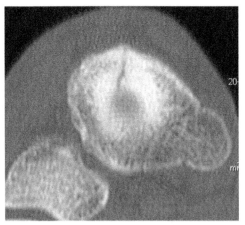

Fig. 5. CT scan image demonstrating a typical fracture pattern of a navicular stress fracture.

Saxena and Fullem[14] created a classification system of navicular stress fractures based on frontal-plane CT-scan findings. They classified fractures involving only the dorsal cortex as type I fractures (**Fig. 6**), fractures that extended into the navicular body as type II fractures (see **Fig. 5**), and fractures that traversed the entire navicular into the plantar cortex as type III fractures (**Fig. 7**).

MRI Scans

Although MRI scan is an exceedingly sensitive diagnostic tool, few articles describe the use of MRI scans in the diagnosis of navicular stress fractures.[12,15] Burne and colleagues[12] compared CT scan and MRI scan findings in their series of 20 navicular stress injuries, including 11 navicular stress fractures and 9 navicular stress reactions. They found that CT scan was more accurate in detecting navicular stress fractures than MRI. There were seven fractures seen on CT scan not noted by MRI, and only

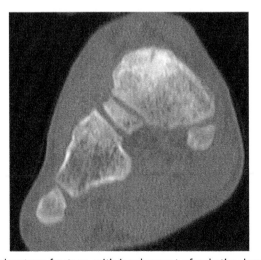

Fig. 6. Type I navicular stress fracture, with involvement of only the dorsal cortex.

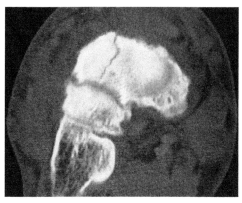

Fig. 7. Type III navicular stress fracture, with extension of the fracture through the plantar cortex.

one fracture detected on MRI that was not seen on CT. Conversely, all navicular stress reactions were, by definition, identified by abnormal signal on MRI, but with no evidence of abnormality on CT scan (**Figs. 8** and **9**). MRI may become more important as increased awareness leads to earlier diagnosis of this injury. Being able to define a stress reaction before it progresses to a stress fracture may reduce the morbidity seen with this injury.

Authors' Recommendation

Plain radiographs of the foot and ankle are the first diagnostic test ordered when there is suspicion for a navicular stress fracture, as much to rule out other pathology as to diagnose a stress fracture. If no clear etiology of the patient's symptoms is identified, a CT scan is then ordered. CT scans have been found to be more accurate than MRI for diagnosing and characterizing a navicular stress fracture. If CT scan is negative,

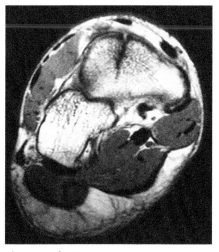

Fig. 8. MRI scan of navicular stress fracture.

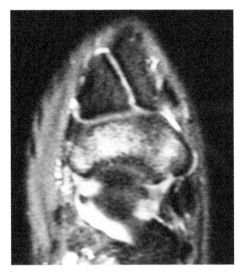

Fig. 9. MRI scan of navicular stress reaction, with extensive edema throughout the navicular, but no fracture line noted.

and a high clinical suspicion persists, an MRI scan is then obtained to rule out a stress reaction in one of the tarsal bones.

DIFFERENTIAL DIAGNOSIS

Because a navicular stress fracture may present with indistinct symptoms, there are numerous other conditions that need to be considered in the differential diagnosis of an athletic individual presenting with midfoot or hindfoot pain. This includes other conditions involving the navicular bone itself, and conditions involving adjacent bones, joints, or anatomic structures (**Box 1**).

A navicular stress reaction will present with identical symptoms to a stress fracture, because it is a nearly identical condition and possibly a precursor to a fracture. The differentiation between the two conditions is increased uptake on a bone scan or signal abnormality on an MRI scan with a negative CT scan. The treatment of a navicular stress reaction is similar to that of a type I navicular stress fracture, with a period of nonweight bearing, followed by protected weight bearing and gradual resumption of physical activities.

A painful accessory navicular usually presents with more localized pain over the medial navicular, at the site that the accessory bone attaches to the navicular. However, because the majority of accessory naviculars are asymptomatic, a navicular stress fracture may be present when an accessory navicular is noted on diagnostic studies. Therefore, a careful physical examination is necessary to determine if the accessory navicular is truly symptomatic or if there may be a stress fracture present as well.

Posterior tibial tendonitis presents with pain along the medial aspect of the navicular that may extend along the course of the tendon up to the medial malleolus. There may be swelling over the tendon, and there is usually pain with resisted inversion of the foot, findings that are usually not be present with a navicular stress fracture.

Tarsal coalitions may present with symptoms similar to a navicular stress fracture. A calcaneonavicular coalition will present with pain over the dorso-lateral aspect of the

Box 1
Differential diagnosis of navicular stress fracture

Conditions involving the navicular bone

   Navicular stress reaction

   Accessory navicular

   Insertional posterior tibial tendonitis

   Calcaneo navicular coalition

   Osteonecrosis of the navicular

   Osteoarthritis of the talonavicular joint

Conditions elsewhere in the foot and ankle

   Stress fracture of other tarsal bones

   Anterior tibial tendonitis

   Talo calcaneal coalition

   Osteochondral defect of the talus

   Talar neck bone spurs

navicular. A talocalcaneal coalition is more likely to present with vague hindfoot pain. Both conditions will demonstrate marked restrictions in subtalar motion. An oblique X-ray of the foot will help identify a calcaneonavicular coalition, but a CT scan is usually necessary to diagnose a talocalcaneal condition.

A stress fracture elsewhere in the midfoot or hindfoot may present with symptoms similar to a navicular stress fracture. This includes a stress fracture of the talus, cuboid, cuneiforms, or even the proximal aspect of the metatarsals. MRI scan will distinguish these conditions from a navicular stress fracture.

Anterior tibial tendonitis is uncommon, and presents with pain at the tendon's insertion into the medial cuneiform or over the distal course of the tendon, which is right over the navicular bone. This condition may be distinguishable form a navicular stress fracture by careful palpation of the tendon, and by a finding of pain with resisted dorsiflexion of the ankle.

Ankle joint pathology may be difficult to distinguish from a navicular stress fracture. An osteochondral defect of the talus or talar neck bone spurs may present with non-localized activity-related pain over the anterior ankle and foot. Plain X-rays of the foot and ankle may help to diagnose either of these conditions, and an MRI scan of the ankle will clearly distinguish them from a possible navicular stress fracture.

Several uncommon conditions affect the talonavicular joint and may present with similar symptoms to a navicular stress fracture. Osteonecrosis of the navicular, osteochondral defects of the talar head, and osteoarthritis of the talonavicular joint will all cause pain around the area of the navicular. Advanced stages of osteonecrosis and osteoarthritis will be distinguishable from a navicular stress fracture on plain X-rays. An osteochondral defect or early-stage osteonecrosis will take an MRI scan to distinguish from a navicular stress fracture.

TREATMENT OF NAVICULAR STRESS FRACTURES

After properly diagnosing a navicular stress fracture, the next challenge is prescribing the proper treatment. Proper treatment will allow for the best chance of timely healing of the fracture, will lower the risk of developing a recurrent stress fracture, and will help to avoid other complications associated with surgical and nonsurgical treatment of navicular stress fractures. However, there is some disagreement in the literature as to the best treatment for navicular stress fractures.

Literature Review

Khan and colleagues'[10] study of 86 navicular stress fractures emphasized the importance of nonweight bearing immobilization for treatment for these injuries. Of the 22 fractures treated with 6 weeks of nonweight bearing, 86% returned to sports, at an average of 5.6 months. Of the 34 treated with limited activity but continued weight bearing for 6 weeks, only 26% returned to sports. Khan also found that in this latter group that failed treatment, if they were then immobilized in a nonweight bearing cast, their outcome was better than surgical repair as a second treatment modality. Khan concluded that the treatment of choice for navicular stress fractures was nonweight-bearing cast immobilization.

In opposition to Khan, Fitch and colleagues[7] strongly recommended surgical treatment of specific types of navicular stress fractures. Fitch's treatment recommendations were based on what he felt was the unpredictable nature of healing of navicular stress fractures, which was detailed with the advent of CT scanning for these injuries. He felt that the fractures would become asymptomatic with initial treatment, but were not necessarily healing, and he found that symptoms would recur once athletic endeavors were restarted. For this reason, Fitch recommended a more aggressive surgical approach to these fractures. His technique consisted of en-bloc resection of the fracture surfaces, autologous bone grafting with corticocancellous block graft, and no internal fixation. Fitch recommended surgical repair of complete or comminuted fractures and incomplete fractures, which extended to become complete or almost complete. He also recommended surgery for fractures with delayed or nonunion fractures with medullary cysts, demonstrated by sclerosis of the cortex, and fractures that did not heal with nonweight-bearing cast immobilization for 8 to 10 weeks. Fitch treated 19 fractures surgically out of the 34 navicular stress fractures in his study.

Torg and colleagues[9] reviewed 21 patients treated for navicular stress fractures in a multicenter study. He found that all 10 fractures treated with a nonweight-bearing cast healed, whereas 7 of 9 fractures treated with weight bearing, whether in a cast or not, failed to heal or the fracture later recurred. Torg recommended treatment of partial or nondisplaced complete navicular stress fractures in a nonweight-bearing cast for 6 to 8 weeks. Displaced fractures and nonunions should be treated with surgical repair with internal fixation or bone grafting, followed by a nonweight-bearing cast until the fracture healed.

Burne and colleagues[12] reported on the long-term follow-up of 11 navicular stress fractures, and correlated the outcome with CT scan and MRI scan findings. Only 3 of the 11 fractures regained normal appearing CT or MRI scan appearance, at an average follow-up of 3.7 years.

Saxena and colleagues[16] studied 22 navicular stress fractures and devised a classification system, described above. He found that the more severe the fracture, the longer the average time to return to full activity. He also found that patients who underwent surgery had a return to activity earlier than patients treated without surgery. Saxena concluded that type II and III navicular stress fractures should undergo surgical repair.

In a second study, Saxena and Fullem[17] reported on the time for return to activity in 19 navicular stress fractures. Patients with type I fractures were treated nonoperatively and had an average time to return to activity of 3.8 months. Type II and III fractures underwent surgical repair, and had an average time to return to activity of 3.7 and 4.2 months, respectively.

In an article comparing the outcome of surgical versus nonsurgical treatment of navicular stress fractures, Potter and colleagues[13] studied 32 fractures, with an average of 10 years of follow-up. Of these, 19 fractures had been treated conservatively and 13 surgically. He found similar function, pain level, and CT findings between the two groups. Of particular interest was that at even 10-years follow-up, some CT scans showed a persistent cleft at the fracture site.

Treatment

The treatment of navicular stress fracture is evolving. The literature demonstrates the ability of these fractures to heal without surgery, albeit with prolonged immobilization and limitation of activities. Because navicular stress fractures are most commonly seen in elite athletes who want to minimize their time away from competition, they might opt for surgical repair of their fracture if it means returning to their sport sooner or with lower risk for recurrent injury.

Furthermore, once an athlete has sustained a navicular stress fracture, they are at high risk of developing a recurrent stress fracture at the same site if they return to their pre-injury level of activity. It makes biomechanical sense that internal fixation of the fracture site will add strength to the navicular, and therefore will likely diminish the risk of re-fracturing the bone.

Authors' Recommended Treatment

Type I fractures are treated in a nonweight-bearing cast for 6 weeks. A fiberglass cast is used for 4 weeks, followed by a removable cast, which can be removed for sleeping and for showering. At the 6-week time-point, weight bearing is allowed in the removable cast, and nonimpact activities, such as a stationary bike, elliptical trainer, water-running, and swimming. At the 8-week time-point, if the patient has been symptom-free walking in the cast, the cast may be removed for all activity. Resistive strengthening exercises can be performed with the foot and ankle. Light jogging on a treadmill can begin at this point, or running on an "antigravity" treadmill, which allows partial body-weight running. By 10 weeks, full running activity can resume and sport-specific training can commence, including agility training. If there have been no symptoms during this time period, full return to sports can be attempted at 12 weeks following the beginning of treatment. If there is some persistent pain, or if this is a recurrent stress fracture, a CT scan should be obtained before full release to physical activities.

Elite athletes, including competitive collegiate athletes and professional athletes, may wish to undergo percutaneous screw fixation of type I navicular stress fractures, to enable them to return to competition more quickly and reduce the risk of a recurrent stress fracture.

Technique of Percutaneous Screw Fixation

The site of the fracture is carefully evaluated on CT scan, as it will not be visible on intraoperative radiography. Under fluoroscan guidance, guide pins are placed across the navicular fracture site. The first pin is placed proximally and dorsally in the navicular. The second pin is then placed parallel to the first, but more distally and slightly more plantar, so it does not interfere with the first screw (**Fig. 10**). The partially threaded screws are placed strategically so that the threads gain as much purchase

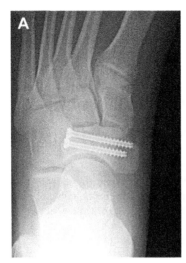
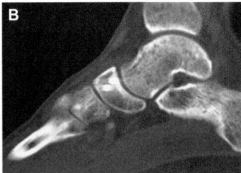

Fig.10. (*A* and *B*) AP and lateral images of proper screw placement for fixation of a navicular stress fracture.

in the larger fragment of bone as possible. This usually means placing the screws from lateral to medial, but it depends on the exact location of the fracture site.

The authors use 4-mm cannulated screws for this surgical technique, either stainless steel or titanium. Smaller screws can be used, but are not as strong and therefore have an increased risk of breakage. Larger screws may also be used, but it may be technically difficult to position two screws correctly in the navicular. Noncannulated screws can also be used; they have the advantage of being stronger but are more difficult to place precisely.

Following surgical repair of a type I navicular stress fracture, a patient is placed in a removable walking cast, nonweight bearing for 4 weeks. Partial weight bearing is allowed at 4 weeks, and at 6 weeks the cast is discontinued and activity is gradually resumed. Running can resume at 8 weeks, symptoms-permitting.

Patients with type II navicular stress fractures are generally advised to have surgical repair of the navicular, especially if there is evidence of sclerosis at the edges of the fracture. The authors recommend directly exposing the fracture site and bone grafting, along with cannulated screw fixation for these fractures. The healing rate appears to be improved and the risk of a refracture is probably reduced following surgical repair. The time-frame to resume athletic activities is shorter following operative treatment.

Technique of Open Surgical Repair with Bone Grafting

The fracture site is approached through a dorsal longitudinal incision, usually over the middle third of the navicular, but depends on the CT scan findings as to where the dorsal cortex is fractured. Careful attention is made during the dissection to not damage the cutaneous nerves or neurovascular bundle. The site of the fracture on the dorsal cortex may be difficult to find, and the CT scan is referred to for guidance. The talonavicular joint is exposed and an arthrotomy is made. This often helps to determine the precise site of the fracture because it usually involves the proximal cortex of the navicular. Fibrous tissue is removed from the entire fracture site by using a small curette, and the distal and plantar extent of the fracture is determined. If there is significant sclerotic bone present, it is removed with a rongeur or curette, back to healthy-appearing bone. The fracture site is drilled with a small drill or K-wire to promote blood circulation to the dorsal cortex of the navicular. If the fracture extends more than 2 mm to 3 mm into the navicular, or if the fracture gap is more than 1-mm to 2-mm wide, then harvesting bone graft is recommended to pack into the bone defect. The graft is harvested either from the lateral wall of the calcaneus or from the distal medial tibia, just above the medial malleolus. Cancellous bone is packed into the fracture site. A piece of cortical bone may also be used to place over the dorsal cortex of the navicular. If the fracture line is small and there is no resorption of the bone edges, there may be no place for bone graft, and therefore bone grafting is not performed.

Once the bone graft has been impacted into place, two percutaneous screws are placed across the fracture site using the same technique as outlined in the section above. After surgical repair of a type II navicular stress fracture, the patient is kept nonweight bearing for 6 weeks, followed by 2 weeks of weight bearing in a cast boot. Nonimpact activity can then gradually resume, but running is not allowed until a CT scan has confirmed healing of the stress fracture, at approximately 3 months.

The treatment regimen for an individual who chooses nonoperative treatment for a type II stress fracture is similar to that for a type 1 fracture up to the 8-week timeframe. Running is not permitted until a CT scan shows evidence of healing of the fracture, and is not allowed before 4 months.

The treatment of type III navicular stress fractures is similar to that of type II fractures. Surgical repair with bone graft and internal fixation is recommended. The postoperative regimen consists of 2 months of strict nonweight bearing, followed by protected weight bearing for another month. At 3 months, nonimpact activities are resumed. A CT scan is obtained at 4 months to assess for healing, before the athlete is released to running activities.

Bone Stimulators

There is no literature that supports the routine use of bone stimulators as an adjunct modality for treatment of navicular stress fractures. Saxena and collegues[16] used a pulsed electromagnetic fields device in 11 patients, and actually noted these patients had a longer time to return to activity than patients not using the device. Lee and Anderson[18] recommend using an implantable bone stimulator when treating nonunions of navicular stress fractures.

Orthotics

The use or avoidance of custom or over the-counter orthotics in the treatment algorithm of navicular stress fractures has not been advocated. This may be because the incidence of navicular stress fractures has never been correlated with a certain foot type, either cavus or planus. In the authors' opinion, when an athlete is returning to competition following treatment of a navicular stress fracture, they should wear a shoe with a supportive arch and should be considered for a semi-rigid custom orthotic, especially in a patient with a cavus arch.

ADVERSE OUTCOMES

The possible adverse outcomes of treatment of navicular stress fractures includes fracture nonunion or delayed union, refracture of a previously healed fracture, persistent pain after treatment, and the development of talonavicular joint arthritis. There are also specific complications associated with surgical repair of navicular stress fractures.

Nonunion and Delayed Union

The rate of nonunion following treatment of navicular stress fractures is difficult to calculate, given the paucity of cases in the literature and the lack of posttreatment imaging studies to adequately confirm healing or nonhealing of the fractures. However, the incidence of nonunion or "treatment failures" appears to be low following both nonsurgical and surgical treatment.

When treated with at least 6 weeks of nonweight-bearing cast immobilization, only 1 of 22 patients treated in Khan and colleagues'[10] series and no patients in Torg and colleague's[9] series of 10 patients developed a nonunion. Saxena reported two apparent nonunions in 13 conservatively treated patients.[16,17] Many other studies do not report the conservative treatment protocols that were used, so it is possible the nonunions or "treatment failures" that are reported did not receive appropriate nonweight-bearing immobilization.

When treated with surgical repair, only 1 of the 19 fractures treated by Fitch and colleagues[7] with bone grafting, and none of Saxena's 22 surgically patients developed a nonunion.[16,17] Three out of five patients in Khan and colleagues'[10] series who had failed previous surgical treatment went on to a nonunion after their second surgical attempt.

In the one study that had CT scan follow-up on all patients, Kiss and colleagues[14] found 12 out of 55 cases developed nonunions. However, Kiss did not describe the treatment regimens for his patients, or how long after treatment the CT scans were obtained.

The rate of delayed union of navicular stress fractures is difficult to calculate, given the heterogeneity of treatment protocols and general lack of appropriate follow-up imaging. The only clear delayed union reported in the literature was by Khan and colleagues,[10] who reported one delayed union in their series, which eventually healed after 18 months.

Treatment of Nonunions and Delayed Unions

Nonunions and delayed unions of navicular stress fractures are treated with surgical repair, whether or not they have had prior surgery. The technique is described in the section on open repair with bone grafting. If previous surgery has been performed, aggressive debridement of the nonunion site is undertaken, and abundant bone graft is placed at the fracture site. If internal fixation was placed, the old hardware is evaluated to see if the screws are tight and in the correct position. If so, they are left in place. Otherwise, they are replaced with new screws.

The postoperative regimen includes 6 weeks of nonweight bearing, 4 weeks in a weight-bearing cast, and resumption of athletics at 4 months, once CT scan confirms healing of the fracture.

Recurrent Stress Fracture

Few recurrent navicular stress fractures are described, making it difficult to identify risk factors for developing a recurrent fracture. In Burne and colleagues'[12] series, 2 of 11 patients with navicular stress fractures sustained a recurrent stress fracture, one at 7 and one at 18 months following treatment. Their original treatment regimen was not detailed. Two of Saxena's 13 conservatively treated patients sustained a refracture during the study period.[16] One of Torg's patients developed a refracture after inadequate treatment.[9]

Many patients present with several months of intermittent symptoms before ultimately being diagnosed with a navicular stress fracture. It is possible that many of these patients may be presenting with a recurrent stress fracture and not a "fresh" fracture. The initial fracture may have healed with a course of relative rest, and then the navicular refractured after resumption of activities. It is also possible many of these injuries were initially stress reactions that progressed to stress fractures. Burne found that seven of nine patients in his series that were diagnosed with navicular stress reaction went on to develop a CT-scan diagnosed navicular stress fracture at later follow-up imaging.[12]

A final possibility is that the recurrent injury may be a stress fracture at a different site as the original stress injury, resulting from a weakened area of bone from internal fixation (**Fig. 11**).

Treatment of Recurrent Navicular Stress Fracture

The treatment of a recurrent navicular stress fracture depends somewhat on the circumstances surrounding the reinjury. If a patient has not been treated with adequate immobilization initially and has sustained a type I injury, then a full 6-week course of nonweight-bearing immobilization should be undertaken. Otherwise, recurrent fractures are treated with surgical repair, as described in the section on treatment of nonunions.

Persistent Pain

If a patient has persistent pain after treatment of a navicular stress fracture, the most likely etiology is incomplete healing of the fracture. Other etiologies of persistent pain include prominent hardware, posttraumatic arthritis of the talonavicular joint, or that the pain is the result of an entirely different cause, detailed in the section on differential diagnosis of navicular stress fractures.

Workup of persistent pain after a navicular stress fracture includes a history of the injury and prior treatment, including the precise length of time the foot was immobilized after the fracture. If surgery was performed, the surgical procedure, including any bone grafting, is important to know. Plain radiographs should be obtained to evaluate hardware position and to rule out other etiologies of the pain, such as talonavicular joint arthritis. A CT or MRI scan is usually necessary as well, to determine if the fracture is completely healed or not. Even with hardware in place, modern imaging techniques can usually be accurate enough to determine complete bony union. If hardware is present, the location of the screws must be carefully evaluated, to see

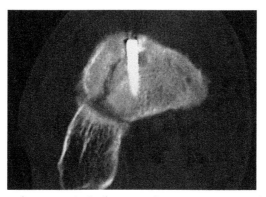

Fig. 11. CT scan image of a new navicular fracture adjacent to a screw used to surgically repair a prior navicular fracture.

if prominent screw tips may be the source of the symptoms. Attention is also given to the cartilage surfaces of the talonavicular joint to evaluate for evidence of arthritis. In addition, the differential diagnosis of other etiologies of midfoot and hindfoot pain must be kept in mind (see section on differential diagnosis).

Talonavicular Joint Arthritis

Talonavicular joint arthritis is a rare but serious long-term adverse event following a navicular stress fracture (**Fig. 12**). Appropriate treatment of a navicular stress fracture, as outlined above, is unlikely to lead to this condition. However, an untreated or neglected stress fracture, resulting in a chronic nonunion, may lead to arthritis. Another cause is osteonecrosis of a portion of the navicular, a rare sequela of a routine navicular stress fracture.

Symptoms of talonavicular joint arthritis may range from a mild, activity-induced aching or stiffness, to constant moderate or severe pain in the hindfoot region. Because the symptoms may be minimal and progress insidiously, the arthritic changes may be quite severe at presentation. The diagnosis is made on plain radiographs, which will show joint-space narrowing and osteophyte formation.

Treatment of talonavicular joint arthritis begins with anti-inflammatory medications and the use of well-supported shoes. A custom, rigid orthotic or University of California Biomechanical Laboratory insert may also help relieve symptoms by adding additional support to the arch. The next line of treatment would be a more-supportive brace, such as an ankle-foot orthosis or Arizona brace. Failing these modalities, the patient is offered surgical reconstruction of the foot. In some cases, a limited debridement of the joint may help, such as removal of dorsal osteophytes. In general, once symptoms have progressed to this level, an arthrodesis is necessary. This can be an isolated talonavicular joint fusion, a double (talonavicular and calcaneocuboid fusion) or triple arthrodesis, depending on the surgeon's choice. Arthrodesis should

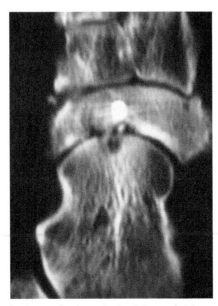

Fig. 12. CT scan image of advanced talonavicular joint arthritis at the site of a previously repaired navicular stress fracture.

be considered only as a last resort. Although it will eliminate the hindfoot pain, all subtalar and transverse tarsal motion is sacrificed, which significantly limits athletic activities.

Surgical Complications

Surgery-specific complications that may occur from repair of navicular stress fractures include infection, nerve damage, and broken hardware.

The infection rate of open or percutaneous repair of navicular stress fractures has not been reported, but is likely less than 1%. Infections can occur at either the surgical repair site or the bone graft-harvest site. Signs and symptoms of infection are no different than at other operative sites. Chronic osteomyelitis following surgical repair of a navicular stress fracture has not been reported.

There are several cutaneous nerve branches than traverse the dorsum of the foot over the navicular. There, branches are at risk for damage at the time of navicular stress fracture repair. The result is a patch of numbness over the dorsal foot or toes that is transient or permanent. Although this will not affect function of the foot, patients find this objectionable and should be warned about this possible outcome before surgery.

Placement of screws across the navicular is a technically challenging task, given the relatively small size of the bone and the goal of placing the threads of two screws entirely within the confines of the navicular. To help make this procedure easier, cannulated screws are generally used. The guide pins of the screws are usually quite small in diameter and are easily broken off in the navicular. Although this rarely presents a problem for the patient, they should be warned of this possibility before surgery. The screws themselves are unlikely to break or loosen. However, the screws may be difficult to remove, especially if the heads strip during attempted hardware removal.

SUMMARY

Navicular stress fractures are becoming more commonly diagnosed because of a higher level of athletic involvement by the population, a greater awareness of the injury, and increasingly accurate diagnostic tools. At least 6 weeks of nonweight-bearing treatment is needed for nonoperative management, usually recommended only for type I fractures. Type II and III fractures are typically treated surgically, often with bone grafting. Gradual return to activity is allowed, with full activity not recommended until a CT or MRI scan shows healing of the fracture. Serious adverse outcomes following treatment of navicular stress fractures have been reported infrequently, but include nonunion or delayed union of the fracture, and refracture of the navicular following complete healing. Treatment of any of these conditions usually requires surgical repair with bone grafting and follow-up imaging studies.

REFERENCES

1. Bateman JK. Broken hock in the greyhound. Repair methods and the plastic scapoids. Vet Res 1958;70:621–3.
2. Towne LC, Blazina ME, Cozen LN. Fatigue fracture of the tarsal navicular. J Bone Joint Surg Am 1970;52(2):376–8.
3. Brukner P, Bradwhaw C, Khan KM, et al. Stress fractures: a review of 180 cases. Clin J Sport Med 1996;6:85–9.
4. Bennell KL, Malcolm SA, Thomas SA, et al. The incidence and distribution of stress fractures in competitive track and field athletes. A twelve-month prospective study. Am J Sports Med 1996;24:211–7.

5. Khan KM, Brukner PD, Kearney C, et al. Tarsal navicular stress fractures in athletes. Sports Med 1994;17(1):65–76.
6. Matheson GO, Clements DB, McKenzie DC, et al. Stress fractures in athletes: a study of 320 cases. Am J Sports Med 1987;15:46–58.
7. Fitch KD, Blackwell JB, Gilmour WN. Operation for non-union for stress fracture of the tarsal navicular. J Bone Joint Surg Br 1989;71:105–10.
8. Golano P, Farinas O, Saenz I. The anatomy of the navicular and periarticular structures. Foot Ankle Clin 2004;9:1–23.
9. Torg JS, Pavlov H, Cooley LH, et al. Stresss fractures of the tarsal navicular: a retrospective review of twenty-one cases. J Bone Joint Surg Am 1982;64: 700–12.
10. Khan KM, Fuller PJ, Brukner PD, et al. Outcome of conservative and surgical management of navicular stress fractures in athletes: eighty-six cases proven with computerized tomography. Am J Sports Med 1992;20:657–66.
11. Pavlov H, Torg JS, Freiberger RH. Tarsal navicular stress fractures: Radiographic evaluation. Radiology 1983;148:641–5.
12. Burne SG, Mahoney CM, Forster BB, et al. Tarsal navicular stress injury: long-term outcome and clinicoradiological correlation using both computed tomography and magnetic resonance imaging. Am J Sports Med 2005;33:1875–81.
13. Potter N, Brukner P, Makdissi M, et al. Navicular stress fractures: outcomes of surgical and conservative management. Br J Sports Med 2006;40(8):692–5 [discussion: 695].
14. Kiss ZS, Khan KM, Fuller PJ. Stress fractures of the tarsal navicular bone: CT findings in 55 cases. Am J Roentgenol 1993;160:111–5.
15. Sanders TG, Williams PM, Vawter KW. Stress fractures of the tarsal navicular. Mil Med 2004;169:8–13.
16. Saxena A, Fullem B, Hannaford D. Results of treatment of 22 navicular stress fractures and a new proposed radiographic classification system. J Foot Ankle Surg 2000;39:96–103.
17. Saxena A, Fullem B. Navicular stress fractures: a prospective study on athletes. Foot Ankle Int 2006;27:917–21.
18. Lee S, Anderson RB. Stress fractures of the tarsal navicular. Foot Ankle Clin 2004; 9:85–104.

Lateral Ankle Instability and Revision Surgery Alternatives in the Athlete

Robert C. Schenck, Jr., MD[a],*, Michael J. Coughlin, MD[b,c]

KEYWORDS

- Ankle instability • Gracilis • Athlete
- Reconstruction • Augmentation

Ankle instability in the athlete is a common problem that is routinely treated nonoperatively, with a 90% success rate.[1–10] With proprioceptive training, preventive equipment (bracing and inserts), and kinetic chain strengthening, surgery for ankle instability is uncommon.[11–13] Prophylactic use of ankle taping and bracing has been shown prospectively to decrease the number and severity of ankle sprains during a sporting season. Nonetheless, some athletes present with recurrent ankle instability that, despite work-up and conservative treatment, requires surgical correction.[14–20] The use of a primary ligament repair (Brostrom procedure) versus augmented (anatomic) reconstructions is discussed in detail in this article.[5,6,21–37]

The work-up for any athlete requires care to evaluate the differential diagnosis of associated injuries such as osteochondral injury to the talus, dislocating or dysfunctional peroneal tendon injuries, and combinations of ligamentous injuries. It is important to clearly define the ligaments involved with an ankle injury. A combination of injuries to the anterior talofibular ligament (ATFL) and the calcaneofibular ligament (CFL) is important in the final determination of the procedure to be performed. The presence of associated syndesmosis, medial deltoid ligamentous injuries, or subtalar instability is also critical in determining appropriate treatment and will be discussed in other articles in this issue. The use of the patient's medical history, physical examination, fluoroscopic stress radiographs, plain films, and MRI can help in determining a clear diagnosis.[38–41]

[a] Department of Orthopaedic Surgery, UNM Lobos, University of New Mexico School of Medicine, MSC 10 5600, 1 University of New Mexico, Albuquerque, NM 87131-5296, USA
[b] Department of Orthopaedics and Rehabilitation, Oregon Health Sciences, 3181 S.W. Sam Jackson Park Road, Portland, OR 97239, USA
[c] Idaho Foot and Ankle Fellowship, 901 North Curtis Road, Site #503, Boise, ID 83706, USA
* Corresponding author.
E-mail address: rschenck@salud.unm.edu (R.C. Schenck).

Foot Ankle Clin N Am 14 (2009) 205–214
doi:10.1016/j.fcl.2009.01.002
1083-7515/09/$ – see front matter © 2009 Elsevier Inc. All rights reserved.

Taking a thorough history for the number and severity of sprains is helpful. The athlete should be asked to provide a visual description of the injuries. In the training room, it is beneficial to ask the trainer and the athlete to describe the mechanism of injury. Athletes frequently provide useful information regarding the position of the foot, the direction of injury, and the location of structures injured. Observing an athlete with a severe chronic instability ambulate in bare feet (especially on gravel) may indicate an ankle that has poor ligamentous joint stability. Furthermore, the type of sport the athlete participates in is important in surgical decision making. Athletes involved in ballet and track and field are best managed with smaller procedures such as a Brostrom/Gould lateral ankle reconstruction. Large athletes with multiple ankle sprains, in the authors' experience, should be considered for an augmented procedure using a gracilis tendon. This is especially important in the presence of joint hypermobility, poor soft tissue and protoplasm, anatomic deformity (such as a varus heel), or a previously failed reconstruction.[42,43]

Lateral ankle instability should first be evaluated by examining the athlete's gait in bare feet before examining the ankle joint. A standard examination should be performed first on the normal ankle to determine range of motion, toe flexion and extension, and associated forefoot and hindfoot abnormalities. Asking the athlete to circumduct the ankle while simultaneously palpating the peroneal tendons for subluxation or pain is useful in ruling out peroneal tendon involvement. The evaluation of peroneal strength as an indicator of adequacy of rehabilitation and nonoperative management is done using resisted ankle dorsiflexion and eversion. The ability to test the ankle for drawer, talar tilt, and subtalar mobility improves with experience. The opposite normal ankle is used as a baseline. The endpoint of the ATFL, CFL, and subtalar joint opening can be further evaluated with a fluoroscopic ankle stress examination.[18–20,38,41]

Stress radiographs may be easily performed by a radiology technician using a specified stress examination protocol with a Telos Stress Device (Metax, Hungen-Obbornhofen, Germany). The fluoroscan has been useful in obtaining stress radiographs. The fluoroscan minimizes radiation to the patient and the clinician. It allows the clinician to carefully assess the subtalar joint for any associated widening. A fluoroscan obtained in the office or training room is less expensive compared with standard digital radiologic imaging.

The authors routinely use a difference of 10° on talar tilt with the ankle held in a neutral position under varus stress in determining a pathologic talar tilt (unstable CFL).[20,38] The anterior drawer should be measured against that of the normal ankle; 10 mm of increased anterior translation compared with that of the opposite side is a useful guide to detect an injured ATFL (**Fig. 1**A, B). The subtalar opening is measured and compared with that of the normal stable subtalar joint. It is still not well defined what degree of radiographic abnormality in subtalar opening confirms subtalar instability.

Although MRI provides good information on ligamentous injury, as seen in other studies in the knee, the use of a clinical examination (especially under anesthesia) is a key part of the determination of a functional ligament. The absence of an osteochondral injury, and the diagnosis of a pure ligamentous injury, leads to a predictable approach to reconstruction for lateral ankle instability. MRI evaluation is critical for preoperative knowledge of an osteochondral injury. MRI is also useful in determining the presence of adequate soft tissues for an imbrication, peroneal tendon longitudinal (split tears) injuries, and evidence of CFL involvement. Thus, an MRI is frequently used in the evaluation of an athlete's ankle instability, but should be used in combination with plain and stress radiographs as well as the physical examination.

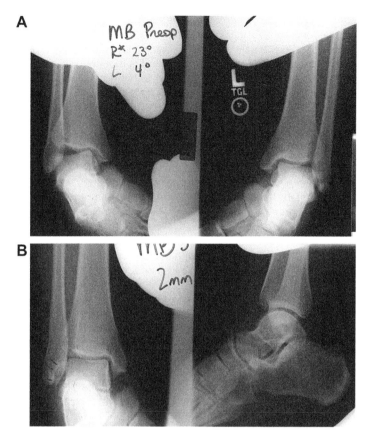

Fig. 1. (A) Stress radiographs showing a significant difference in talar tilt of 23° on the affected ankle compared with 4° on the normal, asymptomatic ankle. (B) Postoperative stress radiographs after an anatomic gracilis reconstruction of the ATFL and CFL showing normalization of ankle position and stability.

For symptomatic patients who underwent previous surgery and present with recurrent instability, it is critical to evaluate them for continued calcaneofibular insufficiency or subtalar instability. Evaluating for available soft tissues, stretched scars, or joint hypermobility[42] also directs the surgeon to the use of an augmented anatomic reconstruction using an ipsilateral gracilis tendon harvest. In athletes with a cavus (or cavovarus) foot and instability, the use of a gracilis augmentation lateral ankle procedure and a Dwyer lateral closing wedge calcaneal osteomy procedure is an accepted treatment approach. If there is a hyperflexed first ray (positive Coleman block test), then a concomitant dorsal closing wedge first metatarsal osteotomy may be included.

SURGICAL TECHNIQUE
Brostrom Procedure

The advantages of the Brostrom procedure are its simplicity, ease of surgery, and size of incision. A small 3-cm incision is made directly over the ATFL in an oblique fashion under tourniquet control. The sharp edges of the ATFL are imbricated with small nonabsorbable sutures, keeping the repair knots small and between soft tissue layers.

The extensor retinaculum has been used and the Gould modification has been per-formed in the presence of CFL insufficiency.[5,6,27,28,44–47]

Rehabilitation following the Brostrom procedure incorporates immobilization and limited weight bearing, with a protection period of 3 months before an increase of activity. There are many studies that demonstrate good functional results with the Brostrom procedure and the Gould modification for associated CFL injuries.

Anatomic Augmentation of the Anterior Talofibular Ligament and the Calcaneofibular Ligament Using a Free Gracilis Tendon

The authors have used this approach for ankle instability in patients with combined ligamentous instability patterns of the ATFL and CFL, associated subtalar instability, large body weight, cavus foot, multiple ankle sprains, inadequate soft tissues, and joint hypermobility (high Beighton score[42]), or for those who require revision surgery (failed Brostrom procedure). The comfort level in this procedure is obtained using a facile approach to the gracilis tendon. The harvesting of this hamstring tendon predictably may require the foot and ankle surgeon to use the assistance of a sports orthopedic surgeon who has experience with the approach and harvest of the medial hamstrings, which is commonly performed with ACL reconstruction. Many different tendon grafts have been used historically; most recently, the gracilis tendon has gained popularity due to its size, ease of harvest, and the minimal long-term disability associated with the harvest.[1,18–21,48–54] Use of an anatomic reconstruction has re-placed the historical tenodesis procedures such as the Evans, Watson-Jones, Chris-man-Snook, and others that have been shown anatomically and in long-term clinical studies to limit subtalar motion.[8,16,17,22,55–63]

In the authors' experience, mistakes in harvesting involve difficulty in isolating the tendon (approach) and amputating the tendon short. The type of anesthetic used in conjunction with this procedure is important. Using a regional sciatic block, the place-ment allows for complete paralysis of the hamstrings to allow for ease of access and harvest. Amputation of the tendon can be avoided by using such a high regional block (sciatic nerve block) or muscle paralysis and general endotracheal anesthesia. Either the block or paralysis allows for ease of traction on the tendon into the exposure. Use of a tendon stripper significantly decreases the possibility of harvesting an inadequate gracilis tendon.[18–20]

The exposure is straightforward, and the tendons can easily be dissected and iso-lated. The pes anserinus can be palpated on the medial border of the tibia, 4 cm below the joint line. The authors typically palpate the tibial tubercle and then place the incision distal and medial to this site, in line with the upper edge of the palpated gracilis and semitendinosus tendons. Although there are reports of use of the semitendinosus tendon, it is too large for most reconstructions of the ATFL and CFL. Paterson and colleagues[49] reported only using half of the semitendinosus tendon. The gracilis tendon is located above the semitendinosus tendon, and after it is identified, the surgeon should ensure that the semitendinosus tendon can be seen below and deep in relation to the gracilis tendon and is not harvested. After soft tissues are released from around the gracilis tendon, the tendon is harvested using a commercially available stripper, and a tendon measuring 15 cm to 22 cm is commonly harvested. The tendon ends are prepared using a locking whip stitch (Krackow-type pattern) and cigar-rolled at the musculotendinous end to make a cylindrical structure at each end. The graft is kept in a moistened sponge and protected in a biopsy cup with a screw-on cap. This allows for maintenance of sterility, even if the cup is accidentally mishandled and dropped.

The surgical approach to the augmentation requires exposure of the fibula and the talar neck, and calcaneal insertion of the CFL. Use of an extensile incision along the fibula that curves anteriorly and distally provides an ease of exposure of the three ligamentous insertion points and the peroneal tendon sheath. This incision is preferred by the senior author of this article (M.J.C.). Another approach is that of the Ollier incision, which is an extended Brostrom or oblique approach to the ankle joint. The incision is marked from the point of the calcaneal insertion of the CFL and half of the distance between the tip of the fibula and the insertion of the ATFL on the talus. This is the incision preferred by the coauthor of this article (R.C.S.). Either approach should be performed sharply, but avoiding injury to the extensor or peroneal tendons. The fibula is sharply dissected to localize the origins of the ATFL (10 mm proximal to the tip of the fibula anteriorly) and CFL (tip of the fibula). The ATFL insertion on the talar neck is easily identified by a ledge of bone just above the sinus tarsi. The CFL insertion is the most difficult to identify and is best approached by going deep to the peroneal tendon sheath (avoiding injury to the sural nerve) and finding the spot 13 mm distal to the talo-calcaneal joint and at an angle 45° posterior to the long axis of the fibula, as described by Burks and colleagues[48] The presence of a previous Brostrom incision must be taken into consideration in the approach to an augmentation, which may simply be lengthened to allow for exposure of the ligamentous tunnel points. After the ankle joint is exposed, the talus is visualized for any osteochondral defects, which are treated appropriately with chondroplasty as indicated. In patients with a failed Brostrom procedure, the imbrication sutures are typically removed, with dependence on the gracilis reconstruction as the sole stabilizer for the ATFL and CFL.

The authors prefer the use of tunnels for placement of augmented grafts, and the drill hole types have been well described elsewhere (**Fig. 2**A–D). Takao and colleagues[52,53] described an interference fixation technique using single limbs of the gracilis tendon. In the technique of tunnels and graft passage preferred by the authors, the length of the gracilis tendon allows for a doubling of tendon grafts, reconstructing the ATFL and CFL with two strands of the hamstring tendon. Furthermore, the cost of biodegradable interference screws is a consideration in addition to the added limb of graft, as compared with the interference fixation technique described by Takao and colleagues.[52,53]

Typically, the authors pass one end of the hamstring tendon through the calcaneal tunnel and suture the tendon to itself. The smaller end is then passed up through the fibula and exits anteriorly, crossing through to the talar neck tunnel. This tendon end is then passed back down through the fibula and routed back into the calcaneus. Each tendon limb is sutured to itself for fixation and tightening of the ligament reconstruction. Wounds are closed in layers before tourniquet release, with application of a bulky Jones dressing and splints.[18–20]

The authors typically change the dressing at one week and place the patient in a well-padded walking boot (Air Cast, Donjoy Orthopaedics, Vista, California), with advancement of weight bearing. At six weeks, the boot is discontinued, and the athlete is allowed to ambulate and perform light jogging as tolerated in an air stirrup (Air Cast, Donjoy Orthopedics). By three months, athletes frequently are able return to sport-specific activities wearing a functional ankle brace.

RECURRENT INSTABILITY AND FAILED RECONSTRUCTION

The patient with recurrent instability after a previous reconstruction is rare when the properly indicated procedure has been performed. In any failed procedure, the surgeon should carefully evaluate the diagnosis and any concomitant abnormalities such as subluxation of the peroneal tendons, the presence of an osteochondral lesion of the talus, or subtalar instability. Certainly, the reported failure rate of the Brostrom

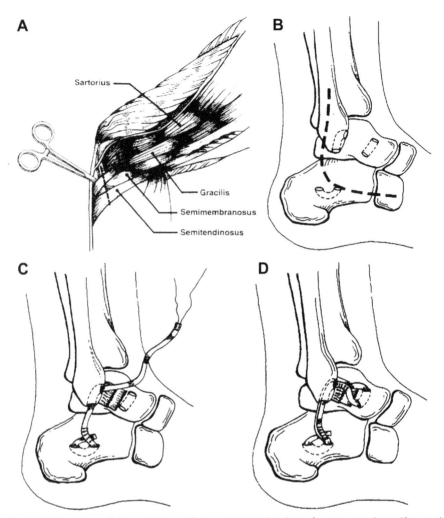

Fig. 2. (A) Exposure of the gracilis tendon at its insertion into the pes anserinus. The semi-membranosus, semitendinosus, and gracilis tendons are also shown. (B) Drill holes made to create tunnels at the origins and insertions of the ATFL and CFL. (C) Starting point for placing the gracilis tendon at the CFL insertion on the calcaneus. The tendon is sutured to itself before passing it up through the fibula, the talar neck, and back through the fibula to the calcaneus. (D) Finished reconstruction with grafts passed and each limb fixed to itself with nonabsorbable sutures. (*Courtesy of* M.J. Coughlin, MD, Portland, OR; with permission. Panel A *from* Coughlin MJ, Schenck RC Jr. Lateral ankle reconstruction. Foot Ankle Int 2001;22(3):256–8.)

procedure is approximately 10%, so it is occasionally observed. In such a scenario, listening to the patient for reports of current problems to determine if there is pain or instability, performing a careful physical examination to rule out peroneal tendon findings, tears, or subluxation, obtaining current stress radiographs to rule out subtalar instability or increased talar tilt, and reviewing a current MRI to evaluate the joint surfaces are four critical areas to confirm to treat what is causally symptomatic. Certainly, an old adage in evaluating any failed reconstruction after the diagnosis is confirmed is to change the procedure and not simply repeat the procedure that was initially performed. The presence of adequate soft tissues, the absence of a cavo-varus foot, or an inherent laxity will often lead to the failure of a Brostrom procedure, and these conditions should be considered as possible causes for the failed reconstruction. In patients with such conditions, the surgeon should consider the use of an anatomic gracilis augmentation as the primary treatment of the instability pattern rather than a Brostrom procedure alone; of course, in the presence of heel varus, a bony procedure such as a closing wedge osteotomy of the calcaneus is indicated.

In the case of a failed Brostrom procedure, the use of an anatomic reconstruction (anatomic augmented reconstruction procedure, as described in this chapter) with an ipsilateral gracilis tendon harvest has been successful in the authors' experience, especially in the patient with inadequate soft tissues or hypermobility. The presence of a cavo-varus foot should direct the surgeon to perform a closing wedge calcaneal osteotomy in addition to the modified Elmslie procedure. Skin considerations with a failed Brostrom procedure are dependent on the previously placed incision. Usually, the use of the previous incision by extending either end will allow adequate exposure of the talar neck, distal fibula, and calcaneus. The surgeon must have a comfort level with the gracilis harvest; without such, the help of a sports orthopedic surgeon with such experience is appropriate.

SUMMARY

In athletes, ankle instability requiring surgery is uncommon. Taping, bracing, and rehabilitation usually allows for 90% of ankle sprains to be treated nonoperatively. In patients who fail nonoperative care, the Brostrom procedure is reliable, cosmetic, and straightforward in its application, with good long-term results. The Brostrom procedure is especially useful in athletes who participate in track and field or ballet and who have straightforward ATFL instability. The authors believe that athletes with a failed Brostrom procedure, subtalar instability, heavy body weight, a cavo-varus foot, ligamentous laxity, calcaneofibular insufficiency, or inadequate soft tissues to imbricate are candidates for an anatomic augmentation of the ATFL and CFL with an ipsilaterally harvested gracilis tendon. With augmentation, athletes can be aggressive in rehabilitation, weight bearing, and eventual return to their sport.

REFERENCES

1. Anderson ME. Reconstruction of the lateral ligaments of the ankle using the plantaris tendon. J Bone Joint Surg Am 1985;67(6):930–4.
2. Ahlgren O, Larsson S. Reconstruction for lateral ligament injuries of the ankle. J Bone Joint Surg Br 1989;71(2):300–3.
3. Barbari SG, Brevig K, Egge T. Reconstruction of the lateral ligamentous structures of the ankle with a modified Watson-Jones procedure. Foot Ankle 1987;7(6): 362–8.
4. Bosien WR, Staples OS, Russell SW. Residual disability following acute ankle sprains. J Bone Joint Surg Am 1955;37-A(6):1237–43.
5. Brostrom L. Sprained ankles. I. Anatomic lesions in recent sprains. Acta Chir Scand 1964;128:483–95.
6. Brostrom L. Sprained ankles. VI. Surgical treatment of "chronic" ligament ruptures. Acta Chir Scand Nov 1966;132(5):551–65.
7. Cass JR, Morrey BF, Katoh Y, et al. Ankle instability: comparison of primary repair and delayed reconstruction after long-term follow-up study. Clin Orthop Relat Res Sep 1985;(198):110–7.

8. Colville MR. Surgical treatment of the unstable ankle. J Am Acad Orthop Surg Nov–Dec 1998;6(6):368–77.
9. Harrington KD. Degenerative arthritis of the ankle secondary to long-standing lateral ligament instability. J Bone Joint Surg Am 1979;61(3):354–61.
10. Nilsonne H. Making a new ligament in ankle sprain. J Bone Joint Surg Am 1932; 14:380–1.
11. Karlsson J, Lansinger O. Chronic lateral instability of the ankle in athletes. Sports Med 1993;16(5):355–65.
12. Prins JG. Diagnosis and treatment of injury to the lateral ligament of the ankle. A comparative clinical study. Acta Chir Scand Suppl 1978;486:3–149.
13. Smith RW, Reischl SF. Treatment of ankle sprains in young athletes. Am J Sports Med 1986;14(6):465–71.
14. Brunner R, Gaechter A. Repair of fibular ligaments: comparison of reconstructive techniques using plantaris and peroneal tendons. Foot Ankle 1991;11(6):359–67.
15. Chrisman OD, Snook GA. Reconstruction of lateral ligament tears of the ankle. An experimental study and clinical evaluation of seven patients treated by a new modification of the Elmslie procedure. J Bone Joint Surg 1969;51A(5):904–12.
16. Colville MR, Marder RA, Zarins B. Reconstruction of the lateral ankle ligaments. A biomechanical analysis. Am J Sports Med 1992;20(5):594–600.
17. Colville MR. Reconstruction of the lateral ankle ligaments. J Bone Joint Surg Am 1994;76:1092–102.
18. Coughlin MJ, Schenck RC Jr. Lateral ankle reconstruction. Foot Ankle Int 2001; 22(3):256–8.
19. Coughlin MJ, Matt V, Schenck RC Jr. Augmented lateral ankle reconstruction using a free gracilis graft. Orthopedics 2002;25(1):31–5.
20. Coughlin MJ, Schenck RC Jr, Grebing BR, et al. Comprehensive reconstruction of the lateral ankle for chronic instability using a free gracilis graft. Foot Ankle Int 2004;25(4):231–41.
21. Elmslie RC. Recurrent subluxation of the ankle-joint. Ann Surg 1934;100(2):364–7.
22. Evans DL. Recurrent instability of the ankle; a method of surgical treatment. Proc R Soc Med 1953;46(5):343–4.
23. Freeman MA. Instability of the foot after injuries to the lateral ligament of the ankle. J Bone Joint Surg 1965;47B:669–77.
24. Gillespie HS, Boucher P. Watson-Jones repair of lateral instability of the ankle. J Bone Joint Surg Am 1971;53(5):920–4.
25. Girard P, Anderson RB, Davis WH, et al. Clinical evaluation of the modified Brostrom-Evans procedure to restore ankle stability. Foot Ankle Int 1999;20(4):246–52.
26. Good CJ, Jones MA, Lingstone BN. Reconstruction of the lateral ligament of the ankle. Injury 1975;7(1):63–5.
27. Gould N, Seligson D, Gassman J. Early and late repair of lateral ligament of the ankle. Foot Ankle 1980;1(2):84–9.
28. Gould N. Repair of lateral ligament of ankle. Foot Ankle 1987;8(1):55–8.
29. Hamilton WG, Thompson FM, Snow SW. The modified Brostrom procedure for lateral ankle instability. Foot Ankle 1993;14(1):1–7.
30. Horstman JK, Kantor GS, Samuelson KM. Investigation of lateral ankle ligament reconstruction. Foot Ankle 1981;1(6):338–42.
31. Karlsson J, Bergsten T, Lansinger O, et al. Lateral instability of the ankle treated by the Evans procedure. A long-term clinical and radiological follow-up. J Bone Joint Surg Br 1988;70(3):476–80.
32. Karlsson J, Bergsten T, Lansinger O, et al. Reconstruction of the lateral ligaments of the ankle for chronic lateral instability. J Bone Joint Surg Am 1988;70(4):581–8.

33. Karlsson J. Chronic lateral instability of the ankle joint: a clinical radiological and experimental study. Medical Dissertation 1989, Goteburg.
34. Karlsson J, Eriksson BI, Bergsten T, et al. Comparison of two anatomic reconstructions for chronic lateral instability of the ankle joint. Am J Sports Med 1997;25(1):48–53.
35. Leach RE, Namiki O, Paul GR, et al. Secondary reconstruction of the lateral ligaments of the ankle. Clin Orthop Relat Res 1981;(160):201–11.
36. Messer TM, Cummins CA, Ahn J, et al. Outcome of the modified Brostrom procedure for chronic lateral ankle instability using suture anchors. Foot Ankle Int 2000; 21(12):996–1003.
37. Nimon GA, Dobson PJ, Angel KR, et al. A long-term review of a modified Evans procedure. J Bone Joint Surg Br 2001;83(1):14–8.
38. Clanton T. In: Coughlin M, Mann R, editors. Surgery of the foot and ankle. 7th edition. St. Louis (MO): Mosby-Yearbook; 1999. p. 1090–199.
39. Kitaoka HB, Alexander IJ, Adelaar RS, et al. Clinical rating systems for the ankle-hindfoot, midfoot, hallux, and lesser toes. Foot Ankle Int 1994;15(7):349–53.
40. Orava S, Jaroma H, Weitz H, et al. Radiographic instability of the ankle joint after Evans' repair. Acta Orthop Scand 1983;54(5):734–8.
41. Rubin G, Witten M. The talar-tile angle and the fibular collateral ligaments: A method for the determination of talar tilt. J Bone Joint Surg Am 1960;42: 311–26.
42. Beighton P, Grahame R, Bird H. Hypermobility of joints. New York: Springer-Verlag; 1983.
43. Inman V. The joints of the ankle. Baltimore (MD): Williams and Wilkins; 1976.
44. Rechtine G, McCarroll J, Webster D. Reconstruction for chronic lateral instability of the ankle: A review of twenty-eight surgical patients. Orthopedics 1982;5: 45–50.
45. Riegler HF. Reconstruction for lateral instability of the ankle. J Bone Joint Surg Am 1984;66(3):336–9.
46. Staples OS. Result study of ruptures of lateral ligaments of the ankle. Clin Orthop Relat Res 1972;85:50–8.
47. Williams JG. Plication of the anterolateral capsule of the ankle with extensor digitorum brevis transfer for chronic lateral ligament instability. Injury 1988;19(2): 65–9.
48. Burks RT, Morgan J. Anatomy of the lateral ankle ligaments. Am J Sports Med 1994;22(1):72–7.
49. Paterson R, Cohen B, Taylor D, et al. Reconstruction of the lateral ligaments of the ankle using semi-tendinosis graft. Foot Ankle Int 2000;21(5):413–9.
50. Sammarco J, Idusuyi O. Reconstruction of the lateral ankle ligaments using a split peroneus brevis tendon graft. Foot Ankle Int 1999;20(2):97–103.
51. Solheim LF, Denstad TF, Roaas A. Chronic lateral instability of the ankle. A method of reconstruction using the Achilles tendon. Acta Orthop Scand 1980;51(1): 193–6.
52. Takao M, Oae K, Uchio Y, et al. Anatomical reconstruction of the lateral ligaments of the ankle with a gracilis autograft: a new technique using an interference fit anchoring system. Am J Sports Med 2005;33(6):814–23.
53. Takao M, Innami K, Matsushita T, et al. Arthroscopic and magnetic resonance image appearance and reconstruction of the anterior talofibular ligament in cases of apparent functional ankle instability. Am J Sports Med 2008;36(8):1542–7.
54. Yasuda K, Tsujino J, Ohkoshi Y, et al. Graft site morbidity with autogenous semitendinosus and gracilis tendons. Am J Sports Med 1995;23(6):706–14.

55. Bahr R, Pena F, Shine J, et al. Biomechanics of ankle ligament reconstruction. An in vitro comparison of the Brostrom repair, Watson-Jones reconstruction, and a new anatomic reconstruction technique. Am J Sports Med 1997;25(4):424–32.
56. Rosenbaum D, Becker HP, Sterk J, et al. Functional evaluation of the 10-year outcome after modified Evans repair for chronic ankle instability. Foot Ankle Int 1997;18(12):765–71.
57. Ruth CJ. The surgical treatment of injuries of the fibular collateral ligaments of the ankle. J Bone Joint Surg Am 1961;43:229–39.
58. Savastano AA, Lowe EB Jr. Ankle sprains: surgical treatment for recurrent sprains. Report of 10 patients treated with the Chrisman-Snook modification of the Elmslie procedure. Am J Sports Med 1980;8(3):208–11.
59. Smith PA, Miller SJ, Berni AJ. A modified Chrisman-Snook procedure for reconstruction of the lateral ligaments of the ankle: review of 18 cases. Foot Ankle Int 1995;16(5):259–66.
60. Snook GA, Chrisman OD, Wilson TC. Long-term results of the Chrisman-Snook operation for reconstruction of the lateral ligaments of the ankle. J Bone Joint Surg Am 1985;67(1):1–7.
61. Tohyama H, Beynnon BD, Pope MH, et al. Laxity and flexibility of the ankle following reconstruction with the Chrisman-Snook procedure. J Orthop Res 1997;15(5):707–11.
62. van der Rijt AJ, Evans GA. The long-term results of Watson-Jones tenodesis. J Bone Joint Surg Br 1984;66(3):371–5.
63. Watson-Jones R. Fractures and joint injuries. Edinburg: Livingston, LTD; 1955.

Osteochondral Lesions: Medial Versus Lateral, Persistent Pain, Cartilage Restoration Options and Indications

Annunziato Amendola, MD[a,b,]*, Ludovico Panarella, MD, PhD[c,d]

KEYWORDS

- Talus • Osteochondral • Cartilage • Lesion
- Repair • Restoration

Chronic giving way and ankle dysfunction are common after ankle sprains (**Table 1**). In a study involving young athletes in 1986, Smith and Reischl[1] reported in basketball players that 50% of the athletes have a dysfunction after sprain and 15% were affected in playing performance. In 1975, Staples[2] described 27% functional instability and 12% sport disability. According to the literature review[3] of more than 100 articles on treatment of ankle sprains, there is a variable (0%–78%) incidence of dysfunction regardless of treatment type: cast, surgery, or functional. In our approach to chronic ankle pain and giving way, one must consider the differential diagnosis before treatment can be directed appropriately.

One of the common diagnoses associated with ankle injury is osteochondral lesions of the talus (OLT). Lippert and colleagues[4] described a 7% incidence of osteochondral lesion after chronic ankle sprains in 962 patients. In 1955, Bosien and colleagues[5] reported on a series of 133 patients; the incidence of osteochondral lesion was 6.7%. The results of acute ankle arthroscopy in a series of acute ankle sprains revealed a medial talar chondral lesion in 66% of cases (30 patients).[6] The advent of MRI also has allowed us to make the diagnosis of occult lesions more readily. In

[a] Department of Orthopaedics and Rehabilitation, University of Iowa Sports Medicine, 200 Hawkins Drive, 01018JPP, University of Iowa, Iowa City, IA 52242, USA
[b] University of Iowa Sports Medicine, 200 Hawkins Drive, 01018JPP, University of Iowa, Iowa City, IA 52242, USA
[c] Knee Surgery, Arthroscopy and Sports Traumatology, Department of Orthopaedic Surgery, University of Rome Tor Vergata, Valle Giulia Private Hospital, Rome, Italy
[d] Department of Orthopaedics and Traumatology, University of Rome Tor Vergata, Valle Giulia Private Hospital, Rome, Italy
* Corresponding author.
E-mail address: ned-amendola@uiowa.edu (A. Amendola).

Foot Ankle Clin N Am 14 (2009) 215–227
doi:10.1016/j.fcl.2009.03.004
1083-7515/09/$ – see front matter © 2009 Elsevier Inc. All rights reserved.

Table 1			
Results of arthroscopic debridement based on diagnosis			
Diagnosis	Procedure	2-Year Follow-up	P value
OLT	3.2 ± 3.1	7.8 ± 3.2	0.0002
Soft tissue impingement	4.3 ± 3.7	8.8 ± 3.4	0.02
Anterior bony impingement	3.1 ± 3.7	7.7 ± 3	0.008
Lateral plica	4.1 ± 2.1	8.7 ± 3.7	0.20
Postfracture scar	3.1 ± 3.3	5.3 ± 3.2	0.14
OA/chondromalacia	2.8 ± 3.3	4.3 ± 3.1	0.31
PVNS	3.7	3.6	NS
WCB	4.1 ± 3.7	4.3 ± 4.1	0.90

Abbreviation: OLT, osteochondral lesions of the talus.
From Amendola A, Petrik J, Webster-Bogaert S. Ankle arthroscopy: outcome in 79 consecutive patients. Arthoscopy 1996;12(5):565–73; with permission.

a retrospective study on 108 ankle sprains, Labovitz and Schweitzer[7] looked at the incidence, location, pattern, and age of occult osseous injuries after ankle sprains. The MRI findings showed bone bruises in 39%. This article discusses OLT, treatment options, and resurfacing techniques.

DIAGNOSIS, INVESTIGATION, AND CLASSIFICATION

Stauffer and colleagues[8] theorized on the correlation between inversion sprains and the increasing of forces applied on the talar dome. With anterior subluxation and inversion of the talus within the mortise, one can speculate how either anterolateral or posteromedial lesions could occur. The diagnosis of OLT is commonly missed on initial examination or radiographs. One must consider chronic pain, swelling, mechanical catching, and giving way possibly coming from an underlying chondral defect. Usually OLT is secondary to trauma, either after a single or repetitive event. The investigation for an OLT may include radiographs, CT scan, bone scan, and MRI to define the location, size, cartilage surface, and joint condition. Posteromedial or anterolateral locations are most common. The sensitivity of routine radiography is 50% to 75%, whereas pickup on bone scan is 99% sensitive. CT scan may be useful for bony anatomy and location of the lesion. MRI is indicated if radiographic results arenormal; it may give information regarding vascularity, healing, and cartilage integrity.

In 1959, Bernt and Hardy[9] classified OLT into four types according to radiographic findings. Canale and Belding[10] classified the lesion into four different types according to the cartilage damage:

Type I: cartilage intact
Type II: partially detached
Type III: complete separation in crater
Type IV: completely displaced in joint

Anderson and colleagues[11] modified the Bernt and Hardy classification according to CT scan findings:

Stage 1: subchondral compression
Stage 2: incomplete separation
Stage 2a: subchondral cyst

Stage 3: detached, undisplaced fragment
Stage 4: displaced fragment

Loomer and colleagues[12] improved CT scan classification by including the type 5 cystic lesions (**Fig. 1**):

Stage 1: subchondral compression (edema)
Stage 2: incomplete fracture, undisplaced
Stage 3: complete fracture, undisplaced
Stage 4: displaced fragment
Stage 5: radiolucent (fibrous) defect, roof intact

Pritsch and colleagues[13] introduced arthroscopic grading:

Stage 1: intact, shiny cartilage
Stage 2: intact but soft
Stage 3: frayed cartilage

The purpose of assessing these lesions is to be able to estimate the size, location, and integrity of the articular cartilage surface to recommend optimal treatment.

Treatment

In the operative treatment of OLT, we need to differentiate between acute and chronic lesions. Acute lesions are usually treated by excision particularly if the fragment is small, displaced, or comminuted (**Fig. 2**A, B). Indications for repair are controversial, but if the fragment is large, repair may be attempted, particularly with an anterolateral location. In our experience, if the lesion is larger than one third of the talar dome width, fixation should be considered. The overall indications for repair can be restricted to the cases of a large lesion (> 35% talar dome surface area) with a cartilage surface intact (**Fig. 3**A, B).

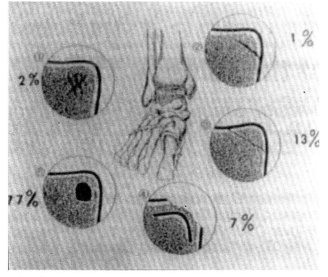

Fig. 1. Loomer classification, types 1 to 5. (*From* Loomer R, Fisher C, Lloyd-Smith R, et al. Osteochondral lesions of the talus. Am J Sports Med 1993;21:13–19; with permission.)

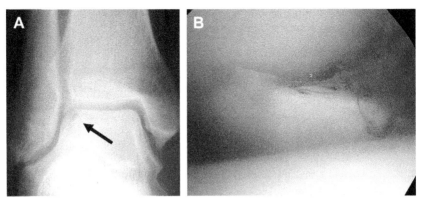

Fig. 2. (*A*) Acute lateral octeochondral fracture after sprain. (*B*) Arthroscopic view before excision.

In chronic types I and type II lesions (undisplaced), multiple drilling versus excision should be considered. Particularly in adolescents, it seems prudent to be cautious with excision and expect a higher rate of healing. In type III and type IV lesions, typically excision or curettage are preferred with predictable outcomes. In Loomer type V, the cystic lesion usually needs to be addressed. Multiple drilling may be helpful, but generally a large cystic lesion may need antegrade or retrograde bone grafting or mosaicplasty. If the articular surface is intact, retrograde techniques are preferred. Usually they are approached though the sinus tarsi under fluoroscopic control (**Fig. 4**A–E). If the articular surface is disrupted, antegrade techniques (ie, mosaicplasty) are recommended (**Fig. 5**A–D). Results of surgical treatment (debridement) are good. Stetson and Ferkel[14] treated 66% medial OLT, 27% lateral, and 7% central. In their series, they achieved 83% good to excellent overall results with debridement. According to various authors and literature review,[15] the procedure has 0 to 90% of good and excellent results.

Amendola and colleagues[16] showed that patients' perceptions of the overall benefit they received from the arthroscopic treatment was best for localized lesions of the

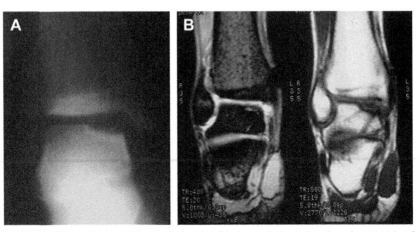

Fig. 3. (*A*) Radiographs in a 16-year-old girl with large (50% talar dome) OLT. (*B*) After fixation and healing, MRI at 6 months.

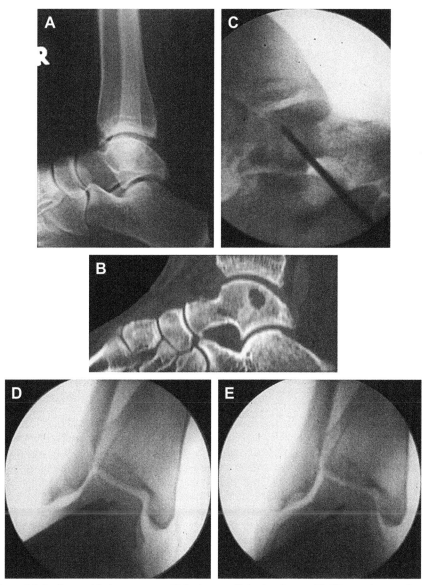

Fig. 4. (A) Radiographic Loomer type V. Lesion medial talar dome. (B) CT scan shows a large cystic lesion. (C) K-wire fluoroscopic positioning. (D) Five-millimeter reamer to enter lesion followed by bone graft. (E) Curettage of the large cystic lesion.

ankle. Outcomes were best for OLT, soft tissue and bony impingement, and lateral plica (outcome based on visual analog scale). More recently, a systematic review of the literature by Tol and colleagues[17] noted that excision with debridement of the bed of the lesion was successful. They showed that nonoperative treatment had 45% success, excision alone had 38% success, and excision and curettage had similar results to excision, curettage, and drilling, with 78% and 85% success, respectively.

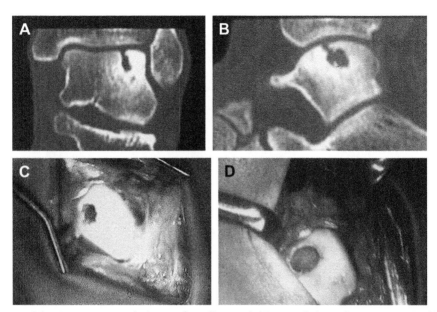

Fig. 5. (*A*) A Loomer type V lesion, surface disrupted. (*B*) Lateral view of Loomer type V. (*C*) Antegrade approach after arthroscopy, anteromedial arthrotomy. (*D*) Loomer type V antegrade grafting.

Posterior Ankle Arthroscopy Technique

In the treatment of OLT, posterior prone arthroscopy[18–20] allows access to posterior lesions (**Fig. 6**A–C). The arthroscopic approach allows for debridement or curettage of the lesion. The exposure to posterior lesions in which resurfacing may be necessary is currently achieved through a posteromedial open approach or a medial malleolar osteotomy (**Fig. 7**). If perpendicular access is required for resurfacing, however (ie, mosaicplasty), then additional exposure can be obtained by arthrotomy with or without a malleolar osteotomy. In a cadaveric study on 11 specimens, Muir and colleagues[21] concluded that 75% of talar dome can be accessed by arthrotomy without osteotomy, that medial and lateral malleolar osteotomies allow 100% sagittal exposure, that anterolateral (chaput) osteotomy[22] provides additional 22% sagittal lateral exposure, and that with all exposures, 15% of residual area is still inaccessible in the posterior central talar dome.

CONTROVERSIES

An asymptomatic finding on radiography/CT/MRI or bone scan remains controversial but at this point is generally left untreated. Posterior lesions—whether posteromedial or lateral—that are difficult to access arthroscopically from a supine and anterior approach need a posterior approach or malleolar osteotomy (**Fig. 7**) or prone posterior arthroscopy (see **Fig. 6**A). Combined mechanical instability and OLT occur often. In general if the symptoms are predominantly pain from the lesion, treatment of the lesion alone is satisfactory; however, if instability is symptomatic, treatment of OLT and instability is necessary. If debridement fails and chronic pain continues after excision, it is necessary to rule out and treat other contributing causes (associated lesions, impingement), treat instability, assess the joint overload at area of lesion, and if

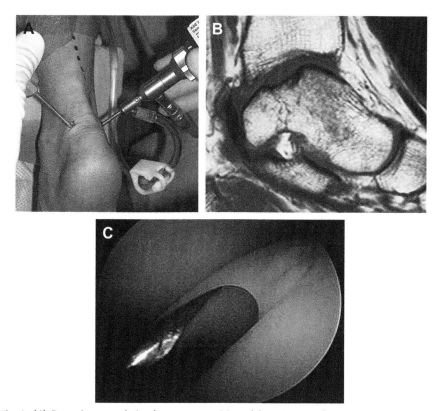

Fig. 6. (*A*) Posterior portals in the prone position. (*B*) Lesion on the posterior downslope better accessed posteriorly. (*C*) Arthroscopic view from posterolateral portal, instrument in posteromedial portal.

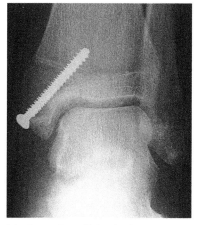

Fig. 7. Operative radiographic step cut medial osteotomy.

present, correct the alignment. If all of the possible contributing lesions have been ruled out, then resurfacing the lesion that already has been treated by debridement may be an option.

Achieving correct limb alignment is most important in any resurfacing or reconstructive procedure. Generally a calcaneal osteotomy—either lateral closing wedge for varus or medial displacement osteotomy for valgus—is the preferred osteotomy. If there is tibial deformity, a supramalleolar osteotomy may be of value. Hindfoot alignment views are essential in assessing overload (**Fig. 8**A–C). If all contributing problems are not present or have been addressed, mosaicplasty or other methods of resurfacing may be indicated. In our experience, the indications for resurfacing are the large lesions (> 1.5 cm) after a failed excision.

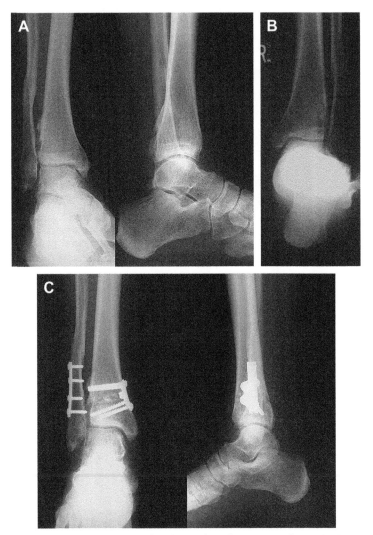

Fig. 8. (*A*) Anteroposterior and lateral radiographis of patient with continuing pain after medial osteoarticular transfer system procedure. Ankle is in pre-existing varus. (*B*) Hindfoot alignment view. (*C*) Postoperative supramaleollar corrective opening wedge osteotomy.

Articular Resurfacing

In general, indication for surgical treatment of these lesions is failure of nonoperative management, in which the patient continues to have symptoms from the lesion despite activity modification, rehabilitation, and bracing. In athletes with acute ankle sprains and displaced osteochondral lesions, one may elect early arthroscopic excision to allow earlier return to play. Indication for articular resurfacing is failure of excision with curettage or drilling. In circumstances in which there is a large bony defect or lesions larger than 15 mm, one may elect a primary resurfacing technique versus excision and debridement.

MOSAICPLASTY

Hangody and colleagues[23] popularized this technique by taking osteochondral plugs from the ipsilateral knee to the ankle. They reviewed 36 consecutive patients with 2 to 7 years of follow-up who were treated for detached lesions larger than 10 mm. Osteochondral grafts were taken from the ipsilateral knee. Malleolar osteotomy was performed in some cases. Postoperatively, patients were managed with 2 weeks of casting (4 weeks with osteotomy). The results were 28 excellent, 6 good, 2 fair. 100% full range of motion was reached by 8 weeks in all cases, and no knee complaints were reported. Others since have reported similar outcomes with few complications.[24–26] The technique has been well described by these authors. Generally they are most commonly indicated for medial lesions.

Athletes who have failed conservative treatment or excision and curettage need further treatment. A medial malleolar osteotomy or lateral chaput osteotomy (the lateral lesions are more anterior) is required. Once the lesions size is determined and the number of plugs determined, either arthroscopic or open procurement of the grafts from the ipsilateral knee is required. My preference is not to take plugs larger than 6 mm from the lateral anterior femoral condyle trochlear ridge (**Fig. 9**A–D). Infrequent donor site morbidity has been reported. Postoperative ankle radiographs show a step off in the subchondral bone plate because the cartilage from the knee is thicker than the ankle.

AUTOLOGOUS CHONDROCYTE IMPLANTATION

The technique of autologous chondrocyte implantation has not had a large experience in ankles of athletes. Often it involves bone grafting ("sandwich"), and malleolar osteotomy is necessary as in the mosaicplasty technique. Nam and colleagues[21] reported 11 cases with 2 to 5 years of follow-up: 9 medial OLT, 2 lateral, 5 autologous chondrocyte implantation alone, 6 autologous chondrocyte implantation and bone grafting. In 10 patients, a second look and screw removal was performed. The results increased from 10 poor and 1 fair (preoperative) to 3 excellent, 6 good, and 2 fair (postoperative. American Orthopaedic Foot and Ankle Society score improved from 47.4 ± 17.4 to 84.3 ± 8.1. MRI and arthroscopy confirmed good fill and improvement from 6 to 24 months. Similar results have been achieved by others.[27–29] Malleolar osteotomy was required in most of these cases using autologous chondrocyte implantation. Giannini and colleagues[28] also used the osteochondral fragment as the source of cells with excellent results.

OSTEOCHONDRAL ALLOGRAFT

Osteochondral allograft transplantation provides mature hyaline cartilage with living chondrocytes with structural support to the osteochondral defect. In contrast to

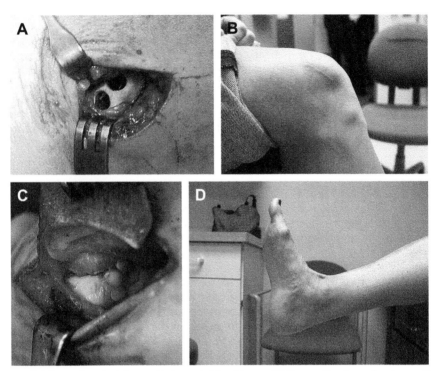

Fig. 9. (A) Osteochondral donor site lateral side of knee. (B) Knee arthrotomy for donor site. (C) Mosaicplasty performed via a mini arthrotomy approach and a medial malleolus osteotomy to treat the lesion located posteromedially. (D) Postoperative clinical picture after medial malleollar osteotomy for osteoarticular transfer system.

autogenous graft from the knee, donor site morbidity is eliminated and this technique allows for restoration of the articular surface by taking the appropriate grafts from the matching donor site. The author's preference is to obtain matched tali, freshly preserved, which gives one the ability to resurface any part of the talar body anatomically, particularly the shoulders (**Fig. 10**A–C). Gross and colleagues[30] initially described fresh allograft transplantation using single talus allografts fashioned to fit into the osteochondral defects in nine patients. Six patients were satisfied with their results and had a mean survival of 11 years. Three patients required ankle fusions. "Fresh" preserved osteochondral allograft was recently described by Tontz and colleagues.[31] Twelve patients affected mostly by bipolar lesions (tibial and talar aspects) with an average age of 43 years were controlled at more than 21 months' follow-up. All grafts healed at the host/donor interface. Complications included intraoperative fracture in one patient and graft collapse that required revision allografting in another. Most patients were relieved of preoperative pain and were satisfied with the procedure; however, there were several reoperations. With newer techniques and improved viability, it is a useful procedure for large focal defects of the talus or tibia. Unipolar lesions expectedly would be more predictable than bipolar. Fresh tibiotalar allografting is an exciting and promising technique in the treatment of articular cartilage defects in young, athletic patients. The major concerns in this procedure continue to be the viability of the cartilage, host-versus-graft disease, and the possible transmission of infective disease.

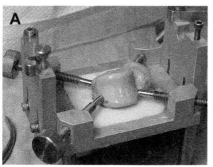
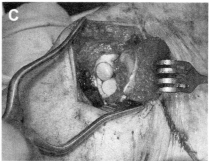
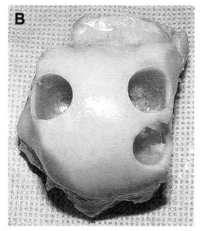

Fig. 10. (*A*) Allograft talus in clamp for preparation. (*B*) Allograft talus presents an anatomic and practical donor for all talar dome lesions. (*C*) Allograft resurfacing medial lesion.

SUMMARY

OLT are a common cause of disability after an ankle sprain. Strategies in management are evolving. Excision and debridement (curettage or drilling) continue to be the mainstay of initial surgical treatment. Articular resurfacing options continue to be popular and continue to improve. The role of autologous or allograft osteochondral resurfacing needs further investigation. For athletes with these difficult lesions, careful evaluation and appropriate operative or nonoperative treatment can allow return to play after 3 to 6 months.

REFERENCES

1. Smith RW, Reischl SF. Treatment of ankle sprains in young athletes. Am J Sports Med 1986;14:465–71.
2. Staples OS. Result study of ruptures of lateral ligaments of the ankle. Clin Orthop Relat Res 1972;85:50–8.
3. Petrik J. The effect of ankle joint effusion on H reflex amplitude. London, Ontario (Canada): University of Western Ontario; 1991.
4. Lippert MJ, Hawe W, Bernett P. [Surgical therapy of fibular capsule-ligament rupture]. Sportverletz Sportschaden 1989;3:6–13 [in German].

5. Bosien WR, Staples OS, Russell SW. Residual disability following acute ankle sprains. J Bone Joint Surg Am 1955;37-A:1237–43.
6. van Dijk CN. Diagnostic strategies in patients with severe ankle sprain. Amsterdam (The Netherlands): University of Amsterdam; 1994.
7. Labovitz JM, Schweitzer ME. Occult osseous injuries after ankle sprains: incidence, location, pattern, and age. Foot Ankle Int 1998;19:661–7.
8. Stauffer RN, Chao EY, Brewster RC. Force and motion analysis of the normal, diseased, and prosthetic ankle joint. Clin Orthop Relat Res 1977;127:189–96.
9. Berndt AL, Harty M. Transchondral fractures (osteochondritis dissecans) of the talus. J Bone Joint Surg Am 1959;41-A:988–1020.
10. Canale ST, Belding RH. Osteochondral lesions of the talus. J Bone Joint Surg Am 1980;62:97–102.
11. Anderson IF, Crichton KJ, Grattan-Smith T, et al. Osteochondral fractures of the dome of the talus. J Bone Joint Surg Am 1989;71:1143–52.
12. Loomer R, Fisher C, Lloyd-Smith R, et al. Osteochondral lesions of the talus. Am J Sports Med 1993;21:13–9.
13. Pritsch M, Horoshovski H, Farine I. Arthroscopic treatment of osteochondral lesions of the talus. J Bone Joint Surg Am 1986;68:862–5.
14. Stetson WB, Ferkel RD. Ankle arthroscopy: II. Indications and results. J Am Acad Orthop Surg 1996;4:24–34.
15. Giannini S, Vannini F. Operative treatment of osteochondral lesions of the talar dome: current concepts review. Foot Ankle Int 2004;25:168–75.
16. Amendola A, Petrik J, Webster-Bogaert S. Ankle arthroscopy: outcome in 79 consecutive patients. Arthroscopy 1996;12:565–73.
17. Tol JL, Struijs PA, Bossuyt PM, et al. Treatment strategies in osteochondral defects of the talar dome: a systematic review. Foot Ankle Int 2000;21:119–26.
18. Phisitkul P, Junko J, Femino JE, et al. Techniques of prone ankle and subtalar arthroscopy. Tech Foot Ankle Surg 2007;6:30–7.
19. Phisitkul P, Tochigi Y, Saltzman CL, et al. Arthroscopic visualization of the posterior subtalar joint in the prone position: a cadaver study. Arthroscopy 2006;22:511–5.
20. Sitler DF, Amendola A, Bailey CS, et al. Posterior ankle arthroscopy: an anatomic study. J Bone Joint Surg Am 2002;84-A:763–9.
21. Muir D, Saltzman CL, Tochigi Y, et al. Talar dome access for osteochondral lesions. Am J Sports Med 2006;34:1457–63.
22. Tochigi Y, Amendola A, Muir D, et al. Surgical approach for centrolateral talar osteochondral lesions with an anterolateral osteotomy. Foot Ankle Int 2002;23:1038–9.
23. Hangody L, Kish G, Modis L, et al. Mosaicplasty for the treatment of osteochondritis dissecans of the talus: two to seven year results in 36 patients. Foot Ankle Int 2001;22:552–8.
24. Al-Shaikh RA, Chou LB, Mann JA, et al. Autologous osteochondral grafting for talar cartilage defects. Foot Ankle Int 2002;23:381–9.
25. Baltzer AW, Arnold JP. Bone-cartilage transplantation from the ipsilateral knee for chondral lesions of the talus. Arthroscopy 2005;21:159–66.
26. Gautier E, Kolker D, Jakob RP. Treatment of cartilage defects of the talus by autologous osteochondral grafts. J Bone Joint Surg Br 2002;84:237–44.
27. Baums MH, Heidrich G, Schultz W, et al. Autologous chondrocyte transplantation for treating cartilage defects of the talus. J Bone Joint Surg Am 2006;88:303–8.
28. Giannini S, Buda R, Grigolo B, et al. The detached osteochondral fragment as a source of cells for autologous chondrocyte implantation (ACI) in the ankle joint. Osteoarthritis Cartilage 2005;13:601–7.

29. Whittaker JP, Smith G, Makwana N, et al. Early results of autologous chondrocyte implantation in the talus. J Bone Joint Surg Br 2005;87:179–83.
30. Gross AE, Agnidis Z, Hutchison CR. Osteochondral defects of the talus treated with fresh osteochondral allograft transplantation. Foot Ankle Int 2001;22:385–91.
31. Tontz WL Jr, Bugbee WD, Brage ME. Use of allografts in the management of ankle arthritis. Foot Ankle Clin 2003;8:361–73, xi.

Plantar Heel Pain

E. Pepper Toomey, MD

KEYWORDS

- Plantar heel pain • Plantar fasciitis • Heel spur syndrome
- Sever's disease • Nerve entrapment

Plantar heel pain is one of the great nuisance pains of the foot and can be a formidable challenge to orthopedic surgeons and other practitioners that manage it. Because it is so prevalent, I have come to call it the "common cold" of the foot. It also tends to behave something like a "cold" in that, no matter what you do, time seems to be as important as treatment modalities. In addition, no one treatment modality has proven itself far superior to others.[1–5] In the 20 plus years of my practice, we have made very little progress on reaching a reliable cure or even knowing the etiology and natural history of this condition. There are a few new treatments, but no particular treatment has come close to being universally successful on its own merit. In reviewing many articles for this article, treatment is always multimodal and even though there is an emphasis on one form of treatment, other modalities are used as an adjuvant to the main modality being evaluated. Therefore, it is extremely difficult to know what consistently works and if one treatment is clearly superior over others.

DEMOGRAPHICS

It is estimated that 1 in 10 people will develop heel pain in their life time. It has also been estimated that 2 million people receive treatment each year for this condition.[6–8] It is rare under the age of 30 and the peak. Incidence occurs between 40 and 60 years of age.[2,3] The factors that seem to be associated with plantar fasciitis are obesity, prolonged walking or standing on hard surfaces, decreased ankle dorsiflexion, and running.[3,9,10] In reviewing articles where surgery was eventually performed, long distance runners comprised a higher percentage than the population at large.[9] There is a slightly higher incidence of heel spurs (75%) in patients with plantar fasciitis versus asymptomatic patients having about a 63% incidence of heel spurs. Despite this slightly higher incidence of heel spurs, it is not felt by most that the heel spur has any correlation to the pain of plantar fasciitis.[11]

ANATOMY

The plantar fascia is a broad ligament originating at the plantar medial aspect of the heel and fanning out to the proximal phalanges of the toes. There are separate bands to each toe that track on each side of the flexor tendons and then insert on the

---

Swedish Orthopedic Institute, 601 Broadway Seattle, WA 98122, USA
E-mail address: etoomey762@aol.com

Foot Ankle Clin N Am 14 (2009) 229–245
doi:10.1016/j.fcl.2009.02.001
1083-7515/09/$ – see front matter © 2009 Elsevier Inc. All rights reserved.

proximal phalanx of each toe. Vertical fibers divide the plantar fascia into three separate compartments connecting to the transverse metatarsal ligament and dermis (**Fig. 1**).[12,13]

The plantar fascia is a relatively inelastic structure. In postmortem studies, maximum elongation is about 4% of the structure and a force of approximately 1000 N is required to failure.[14] The origin at the heel seems to be the most common weak link in the chain of this very stiff structure bearing high tensile forces with the windlass mechanism. This appears to be further exacerbated as result of the gastrocnemius-soleus muscles contracting in the push off phase of gait while the body weight is on the forefoot and the plantar fascia is under tension.

For my patients, I tell them that the bones of their arch are a bow and the bowstring is the plantar fascia. This seems to help in the understanding of the process and what we are trying to accomplish with stretching exercises, eliminating impact activities, and avoiding activities where there is a lot of single limb stance (**Fig. 2**).[13,15] In addition to the plantar fascial anatomy, the clinician must also be aware of the anatomy of the rest of the heel. The fat pad is a closed cell structure containing many septa filled with fat providing a shock absorbing function. The fibrous septa are anchored to the skin and calcaneus resisting shear forces as they also absorb shock. At approximately age 40, there is some fat atrophy and reduced ability to absorb shock.

The other important area of pain is the medial and lateral plantar nerves. Baxter and Pfeffer[16] and Baxter and Thigpen[17] elaborated on this and demonstrated how the first branch of the lateral plantar nerve (FBLPN) becomes entrapped as an etiology of heel pain. They also looked at a series of patients where decompression of the nerve was done with good success.

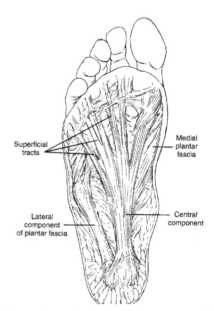

Fig. 1. Anatomy of the plantar fascia. (*From* Myerson M. Foot and Ankle Disorders. Vol. 2. W.B. Saunders; 2000. p. 837; with permission.)

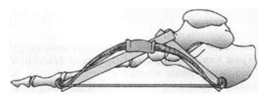

Fig. 2. Concept of the arch being a bow and the plantar fascia a bowstring. (*From* Lee TH, Maurus PB. Plantar heel pain. In: Coughlin MJ, Mann RA, Saltzman CL, editors. Surgery of the foot and ankle. 8th edition. Philadelphia, PA: Mosby Elsevier; 2007. p. 690.)

ETIOLOGY

The etiology of plantar fasciitis is unknown. Early investigators in the 1930s proposed an infectious etiology such as TB and venereal disease prevalent at the time.[18] DuVries[19] focused on the concept of impingement as the result of the heel spur. Cadaveric specimens later demonstrated that the heel spur is at the origin of the flexor digitorum brevis and not at the plantar fascial origin. From a pathologic standpoint, plantar fasciitis is a fibro-fatty degeneration of the plantar fascial origin with micro tears in the fascia and collagen necrosis.[20] Therefore, plantar fasciitis is probably more of a degenerative process rather than an inflammatory process unless the patient has an underlying spondyloarthropathy. Again, plantar fasciitis is associated with obesity, prolonged standing and walking on hard surfaces, running and high-impact activities, and inflammatory arthritis that effect the enthesis such as ankylosing spondylitis. The clinician should especially be concerned about a spondyloarthropathy in patients who are younger than the typical age range and have bilateral heel pain.[12]

In addition to the term plantar fasciitis, this condition is also called "heel spur syndrome." Even though the incidence of a heel spur is higher in patients with plantar fasciitis, it needs to be emphasized that the heel spur is not the cause of the pain. However, once patients are told they have "heel spur syndrome" and see one on x-ray, they often times think they need surgery and will not be well until the spur is removed. Therefore, I discourage the use of this term (**Fig. 3**).

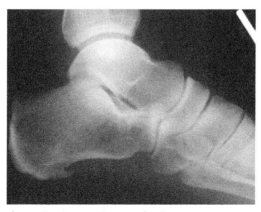

Fig. 3. Do not draw the patient's attention to a heel.

PRESENTATION AND DIFFERENTIAL DIAGNOSIS

The diagnosis of plantar heel pain is based on clinical history and examination. For plantar fasciitis, patients usually have pain directly at the plantar fascial origin at the plantar medial aspect of the heel. They are worse upon arising and improve with stretching and walking. If they sit midday for any prolonged period, they will usually have another episode of pain until the plantar fascia gets stretched out. If their job requires prolonged standing on their feet, I find they are better for awhile during the day but seem to have increasing pain as the day goes on. The pain is nonradiating and parathesias are not common. If a patient has parathesias, the clinician needs to consider nerve entrapment (**Fig. 4**). Patients with tarsal tunnel syndrome will have radiating pain into the plantar aspect of the foot, a positive Tinels sign over the posterior tibial nerve, and a possibility of changes in nerve conduction tests (NCT). However, a negative NCT does not exclude tarsal tunnel syndrome.[16] Those patients with compression of the FBLPN cannot be diagnosed with NCT. Pfeffer demonstrated slightly different areas of tenderness for plantar fasciitis versus entrapment of the FBLPN.[16] I personally have difficulty differentiating between these two conditions but have found the patients with entrapment of the FBLPN to have a Tinel's sign directly over the nerve.

The need to do a "squeeze test" on every patient who presents with heel pain is important. The clinician does this by squeezing the entire tuberosity of the heel to determine if it causes moderate to severe pain. When this is present, I usually find a stress fracture (**Fig. 5**).

Other entities that need to be considered in the differential are L5-S1 radiculopathy, peripheral neuropathies, infection, tumors, tendonitis of the flexor hallucis longus, or other medial flexors of the ankle, fat-pad atrophy.

IMAGING STUDIES

If the patient presents with the typical heel pain of plantar fasciitis, routine x-rays of the heel are not needed. Levy and colleagues[21] evaluated the benefit of radiographic evaluation and found no real benefit in diagnosis or treatment in patients with plantar heel

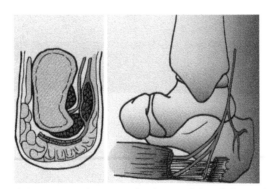

Fig. 4. Entrapment of the FBLPN is between the fascia of the abductor hallucis and medial head of the quadratus plantae muscle. The nerve travels dorsal to the plantar fascia. (*From* Lee TH, Maurus PB. Plantar heel pain. In: Coughlin MJ, Mann RA, Saltzman CL, editors. Surgery of the foot and ankle. 8th edition. Philadelphia, PA: Mosby Elsevier; 2007. p. 690; with permission.)

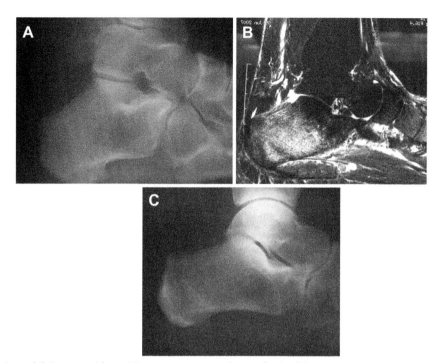

Fig. 5. (*A*) Runner with positive squeeze test at day 5 of pain. (*B*) T2 MRI scan showing stress fracture. (*C*) X-ray finally became positive at week 4.

pain. Unless the patient has a very unusual presentation or is showing no sign of improvement after 2 months of treatment, I do not do an x-ray.[17]

A triple-phase bone scan can be done and is helpful in differentiating plantar fasciitis from a heel stress fracture. Depending on the pathology, patients will show uptake at the plantar facial origin versus a diffuse uptake of the entire tuberosity of the calcaneus.

Bone scans have probably given way to MRI for evaluation. MRI findings of plantar fasciitis include thickening, edema, and increased signal intensity in the substance of the plantar fascia. MRI is probably the best tool to rule out other pathology around the heel and is especially good if a heel stress fracture is suspected. Ultrasonography has also been used and is thought to be as effective as MRI and bone scan for the diagnosis of plantar fasciitis but not other entities around the heel.[21–25]

Unless the patient is not improving or the presentation is unusual, there is no need to start ordering any of these studies on a routine basis for every patient presenting with plantar heel pain.

NONSURGICAL TREATMENT MODALITIES

It needs to be emphasized that nonoperative treatment is the mainstay in treating plantar fasciitis. With time and a good conservative treatment plan, well over 90% of patients will have their condition resolve or reach a tolerance level where it does not have much effect on their lifestyle. There is an exhaustive list of treatments for plantar fasciitis and one only has to look at the Internet to learn about the many modalities and "gizmos" sold to treat this problem. We will discuss the modalities that have been shown to have merit in the literature.

Stretching exercises have traditionally been a primary modality of treating plantar fasciitis. Porter and colleagues[26] reviewed intermittent stretching of the Achilles versus a sustained stretch. Improving dorsiflexion of the ankle over a 4-month period highly correlated with improvement in symptoms and foot function. Both groups improved their heel pain and there was no difference in the outcome with two different methods of Achilles stretching. DiGiovanni and colleagues[27] prospectively reviewed a series of patients who had either an Achilles stretching program or a plantar fascia–specific stretching program. They found both groups improved; however, there was a definite superiority in favor of the plantar fascia–specific stretching protocol. At a 2-year follow-up, 92% of the patients reported total satisfaction or satisfaction with minor reservation.

The idea of stretching or keeping things stretched out has followed with the use of night splints. Theoretically, night splints prevent shortening of the plantar fascia during long periods of rest, thus preventing the initial excessive stretch placed on the fascia upon arising. Wapner and Sharkey[28] reported on the use of night splints in patients who had failed a multitude of other conservative treatment modalities at 1 year. Fourteen patients with 18 symptomatic heels were treated using a night splint in 5 degrees of dorsiflexion and continuing with shoe modification, nonsteroidal anti-inflammatory drugs (NSAIDs), and stretching. Eleven patients had complete resolution within 4 months of treatment. Powell and colleagues[29] also demonstrated the effectiveness of night splints as an isolated modality for 1 month with substantial improvement in 80% of the patients.

NSAIDs are routinely used for plantar fasciitis but their specific value has been looked at in only one study. Donley and colleagues[30] prospectively reviewed 29 patients who were treated with heel cups, stretching exercises, and night splints in addition to being randomized into a placebo group versus a cox-2 (celebrex) group. Pain and disability improved in both groups and there was no statistical difference in the two groups at 1, 2, and 6 months. Subjectively, the investigators felt there was more of a trend for the cox-2 group to do better at 2- and 6-month follow-up. No study has looked at NSAIDs as an isolated entity and there is no good data whereby these drugs can strongly be recommended in the treatment of plantar heel pain.

Orthosis and heel cups have also been one of the primary forms of treatment for plantar heel pain. Pfeffer and colleagues[31] did a prospective randomized 15-center study comparing five groups of patients. Four of the groups received some type of shoe insert along with a stretching protocol and the fifth group did stretching exercises only. All groups improved but the group with a prefabricated silicone insert had the best success (95%) and the group with the custom insole improved the least (68%). Their conclusion was that a prefabricated insole was more likely to produce improvement in symptoms as part of the initial treatment of proximal plantar fasciitis than a custom polypropylene orthotic device. All patients who had a job of prolonged standing were less likely to do well indicating a need for rest in addition to shoe inserts and stretching.[31,32]

Corticosteroid injections have also been popular in the management of plantar fasciitis as well as nerve entrapment syndromes. In a study of 253 orthopedic surgeons, 170 used steroid injections for heel pain. Corticosteroids appear to work early on but it is in question if patients receive long-term relief.[33] Miller and colleagues[34] reviewed 24 patients (27 heels) injected with lidocaine and betamethasone and followed for 5 to 8 months. Ninety-five percent improved with good to excellent relief within the first few days but only 41% felt this level of benefit was sustained. Two important potential complications exist with corticosteroid injections. These are plantar fascial rupture and fat pad atrophy.[65] When injecting the plantar fascia, it is imperative that the injection goes deep and preferably just superior to the plantar fascial origin and not superficially placed anywhere in the fat pad (**Fig. 6**). I do this from a medial approach. In evaluating patients with plantar fascial rupture, Acevedo and Beskin[35] found 44 of 51 patients previously had a steroid injection. Sellman[36] reviewed 37 patients with presumed rupture from steroid injections. All patients had relief of their plantar fascial symptoms but had a variety of new foot problems with flattening of the arch on the effected side after plantar fascial rupture. Most patients resolved their new symptoms with orthotics and other conservative measures but took anywhere from 6 to 12 months to fully recover.

Among its other uses, Botox has been evaluated for the treatment of plantar fasciitis. Babcock and colleagues[37] did a randomized placebo-controlled study of 27 patients (43 feet) using botulinum toxin A. This study showed statistically significant improvement in relief of pain and overall foot function at 3- and 8-week intervals. Placzek and colleagues[38] reviewed nine patients with an average of 14 months of symptoms. Two hundred units of BTX-A was injected into the plantar fascia. Pain was reduced by 50% by 6 weeks and the effect persisted to the 14-week interval. All patients were satisfied enough with their outcome that they did not require further treatment.

Low-dye taping has also been a treatment modality popularized most by podiatry and physical therapy. This technique was first recommended by Dr. Ralph Dye,[39] a podiatrist, who started use of this technique for conditions of excessive pronation. In reviewing orthopedic foot and ankle articles, there has been very little written about this technique and no blinded placebo-controlled study looking at this as an isolated treatment has been done. Scranton and colleagues[40] looked at a gait analysis of patients when they were barefoot versus those with low-dye taping. They found the taping diminished the duration of forces under the midfoot and warranted further study. Radford and colleagues[41] did a randomized comparison of sham ultrasound

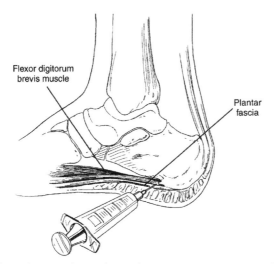

Flexor digitorum brevis muscle

Plantar fascia

Fig. 6. Injection done deep to plantar fascia. (*From* Myerson M. Foot and Ankle Disorders. Vol. 2. W.B. Saunders; 2000. p. 837; with permission.)

and low-dye taping. The participants treated with low-dye tapping had less first-step pain, otherwise there was no difference. Good evidence-based studies on the merits of this technique are lacking.

I have used this technique and followed the guidelines of the podiatry articles for a guide on the technique of taping. There does not appear to be one universal method. I therefore have developed my own technique for athletes. The objective of this technique is to support the transverse and longitudinal arches of the foot and take stress off the plantar fascia.

If I do low-dye taping for an athlete, I use standard 3M athletic tape and the 3M Microfoam tape. I first apply strips from the posterior edge of the heel to the level just past the metatarsal heads. This is done with the Microfoam tape. This tape provides great protection from the cutting and shearing forces of the athletic tape. Once I have about four longitudinal strips from medial to lateral, I will apply athletic tape both circumferentially around the arch as well as strips that start plantar medial and wrap around the heel and then back onto the plantar surface of the foot. I usually leave the tape on for about 4 days and then change it. I have found it more useful in athletes with plantar fasciitis and a tendency to over-pronate (**Fig. 7**).

In the very refractory patient, casting appears to have good benefit. It keeps the plantar fascia stretched out and also induces the best compliance for a period of rest of the fascia. Gill and Kiebzak[1] in a review of 11 different conservative modalities of treatment found casting to be the most effective and Tuli's heel cups the least effective form of conservative treatment. Tisdel and Harper[42] reviewed a series of 32 patients who had been symptomatic for an average of 1 year and had failed various methods of treatment other than casting. Patients were then placed in casts for an average of 6 weeks; 42% of the patients were completely satisfied, 12% were satisfied with reservation, and 46% were dissatisfied. Casting therefore appears to be a reasonable option for recalcitrant plantar fasciitis.[43]

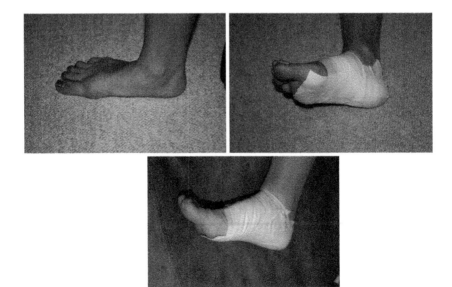

Fig. 7. Low-dye taping: Strips of 3M Microfoam tape are applied across the longitudinal arch followed by strips of athletic tape as shown above.

Extracorporeal shock wave therapy (ESWT) is the newest noninvasive form of treatment for plantar fasciitis. Based on lithotripsy technology, shock waves are used to break up scar tissue and induce neovascularization of the area. There are both high-energy and low-energy units based on the focus energy density (mL/mm^2). All units create shock waves by converting electrical energy into mechanical energy in a water medium. Current indications for ESWT are pain that has lasted at least 6 months and recalcitrant to three or more conservative modalities. There have been numerous articles and all seem to have moderate success.[44–48] It must be remembered that this modality is used only on patients who are refractory to all other conservative treatments. Ogden and colleagues[49] did a meta-analysis of eight separate articles involving 840 patients. Success rates were as high as 88%. It was their feeling that this should be tried before surgical intervention. The authors also felt it was a very safe treatment and probably safer than a steroid injection that could lead to plantar fascial rupture. The only problem I have encountered with ESWT is cost. The cost of a single treatment is about $1100 in the Pacific Northwest and I have been refused payment by four different insurance carriers. These have all been patients who have had plantar fasciitis for at least 6 months and tried all other options.

SURGERY

Because the natural history of plantar fasciitis is not really known, all authors feel surgery should not be considered before 6 months to a year of conservative treatment. With the advent of endoscopic plantar fascial release, the American Orthopaedic Foot & Ankle Society (AOFAS) came out with a position statement stating that all patients should receive 6 months of conservative treatment before surgery is considered.[2] All surgical procedures entail a partial release of the plantar fascia. If the release is done endoscopically, release of the FBLPN is not possible in a reliable manner.[16] Therefore, if the patient has nerve compression symptoms, an open release of the nerve and partial release of the fascia with heel spur excision is advised.

The outcome of open surgery has been relatively good in multiple series. Leach and colleagues[50] reviewed 14 athletes (15 heels) who failed conservative treatment for 1 year. The patients all underwent plantar fascial release with a small sliver of bone removed as well to remove any spur. All patients returned to athletics and only one patient did not improve to their previous level of competition. Three world-class marathon runners were included in this group. There were no complications. Watson and colleagues[51] reviewed patients treated with a distal tarsal tunnel release and partial plantar fasciotomy. Overall, 91% of the patients were somewhat to very satisfied with their outcomes. Baxter and Pfeffer[16] reviewed 69 heels in 53 patients with chronic heel pain emphasizing release of the FBLPN. Sixty-one heels had excellent or good results and 57 heels had complete resolution of pain. Four heels required additional surgery for persistent pain. Additional complications included two postop neuromas, two superficial wound infections, and one with a mild dystrophy. Sammarco and Helfrey[52] followed a series of 26 patients (35 feet) treated with partial plantar fascial release and release of the FBLPN. Thirty-two (92%) had a satisfactory outcome and three (8%) had an unsatisfactory outcome. There were four complications including two superficial infections, one superficial phlebitis, and one deep vein thrombophlebitis.[52,53] Besides these complications that are somewhat common to any foot surgery, the only unusual complication I found was stress fracture after excessive spur removal as reported by Manoli and colleagues.[54] This occurred in four patients with excessive spur removal.

Endoscopic plantar fascial release has the advantage of being minimally invasive. The only other real advantage of this technique appears to be recovery time. Kinley and colleagues[55] compared 66 endoscopic plantar fascial releases to 26 patients done with an open technique. On an average, the endoscopic group returned to activities at 6.3 weeks and the open group at 10.3 weeks. Complications of neuritis, recurrent pain, and infection occurred in both groups but was higher (41%) in the endoscopic group versus 35% percent in the open group. Brekke and Green[56] reviewed 44 patients (54 procedures) who were treated with open release (24 patients), endoscopic release (13 patients), and a minimal incision technique (7 patients). Patients rated as satisfied were 78.8% in the open group, 67.7% in the endoscopic group, and 71.4% in the minimal incision group. The time for recovery to normal activities was about 5 weeks faster in the endoscopic group versus the other two groups.

Release of the plantar fascia is not a benign procedure for the foot. Sharkey and colleagues[57] did a cadaver model where the foot was loaded and portions of the plantar fascia were divided. Cutting the medial half of the plantar fascia increased the pressure under the metatarsal heads. When the fascia was completely divided, strain at the dorsal aspect of the second metatarsal increased by 80%. Thordarson and colleagues[58] showed that by sequentially releasing the plantar fascia in 25% increments, arch height consistently decreased. Daly and colleagues[59] reviewed 13 patients (16 feet) who had follow-up from 4.5 to 15.0 years following central release of the fascia. The longitudinal arch was flattened and abnormalities of foot function persisted. Seventy-one percent of the patients were happy with their outcome. Brekke and Green also emphasized the need to release only the medial third of the fascia when doing an endoscopic release.[56] Gormley and Kuwada[60] had 94 patients who underwent a more extensive open plantar fascial release. At least 50% of the patients reported lateral foot pain that they felt resolved in most patients.[61] It appears there is now agreement in both the orthopedic and podiatric literature that complete plantar fascial release should not be done for fear of causing a lateral column syndrome.[12] Patients develop midfoot pain and pain over the lateral aspect of the foot from excessive plantar fascial release and loss of the windlass mechanism. This causes compressive forces to develop in the midfoot and the lateral side of the foot with a progressive flattening of the arch.

When reviewing plantar heel pain in athletes, it is necessary to discuss Sever's disease. This is an inflammation of the calcaneal apophysis that appears between 4 and 7 years in girls and 7 to 10 years in boys. Multiple centers of ossification show up initially and they gradually coalesce to form one apophyseal center that later unites with calcaneus at 12 to 15 years of age. Sever[62] described the condition in patients who were overweight, physically active, and strong. He recommended a cushion or rubber pad for the heel.

Ferguson and Gingrich[63] studied radiographs of 100 children looking at the calcaneal apophysis. It was usually less dense and irregular than the surrounding bone. An irregular sclerotic physis was the rule rather than the exception.

Scharfbillig and colleagues[64] did a literature review on Sever's disease and found respected opinions prevailed over evidence-based studies on what is really known about this condition (**Fig. 8**).

The patients I have treated for this have nondiagnostic radiographs and clinical findings make the diagnosis. The patients are not a particular body type but the number one sport is soccer. Over 80% of the patients in my practice with this are male. They have a positive squeeze test as the most reliable finding identical to the adult with a calcaneal stress fracture. Most have to take a week off of running to get the

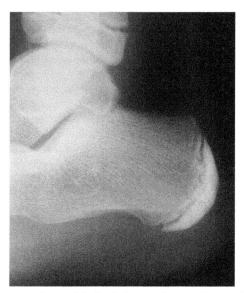

Fig. 8. A 13-year-old soccer player with classic Sever's disease. One week of rest and silicone heel cups got him back to playing for the rest of the season.

apophysitis to settle down but respond quickly to rest. The Silipos heel cup that I condemn later in this article for plantar fasciitis has worked extremely well for this condition. I usually have the patient continue with the heel cup for 2 months after the condition has settled down. I also have athletes use the heel cup on the asymptomatic side so they do not have secondary complaints develop with a leg length inequality. In review of the literature as well as my practice, I have found nothing that shows this apophysitis going on to a Salter 1 fracture or an osteochondrosis of the calcaneal physis.

HOW I TREAT PLANTAR FASCIITIS

When a patient presents to my office with plantar fasciitis, I take a history to learn the onset, duration of the problem, activity level of the patient, location of the pain, and shoe wear. In discussing footwear, the first thing I ask about is going barefoot. After treating a few thousand cases in 20 years of practice, I have had very little success with patients who insist on going barefoot. I tell my patients they must wear shoes even in the house and that very soft slippers without any support are not acceptable. Shoes with a good sole provide shock absorption to the heel as well as decreasing the repetitive stretch to the plantar fascia.

If the patient does not have pain at the plantar medial aspect of the heel, I immediately become suspicious of some other cause as outlined in the differential above. Be especially aware of patients who have pain from a "squeeze test" of the entire heel as they probably have a stress fracture. I have found most patients have a negative x-ray of the calcaneus for the first few weeks with a stress fracture and some never really have significant radiological findings. Therefore, I go directly to MRI scanning if there is a question of another process other than plantar fasciitis, as I feel this will give me the greatest sensitivity for any other pathology including stress fracture. If the patient has symptoms of nerve entrapment, I will get an MRI and nerve conduction test (NCT) early on to rule entities such as a ganglion cyst, bone spurs, tumor, or some other entity causing nerve compression.

A thorough foot examination is completed. On examination, I first check ankle range of motion (ROM) with the knee flexed and the knee straight (Silverskold test). If the patient has a tight Achilles or isolated gastrocnemius equinus, I really emphasize an Achilles stretching program. In discussing a stretching program, I tell patients to first grab their toes and stretch the plantar fascia before they get out of bed (**Fig. 9**).

Then I have them do the Achilles stretch as a separate exercise. I like the Achilles stretch done with the foot flat and not hung over a stool or step as I feel it puts too much force on the fascia. I discuss stretching both the gastrocnemius and the soleus muscles (**Fig. 10**).

Next, I look at the foot configuration. If patients have a significant cavus component to their foot, I think a custom soft or semi-rigid orthotic is appropriate early on. In patients with pes planus I have had better luck with a soft accommodative device that I will later mention. Once I have established the diagnosis and reviewed any contributing pathology, I will start treatment. I do not feel radiographs are needed on the first visit. I want to emphasize that treatment is always multimodal. No single entity works for plantar fasciitis. I first try a three-quarter silicone insole as it works well and will fit in most all shoe wear including dress shoes. A three-quarter silicone insole has consistently worked better than heel cups for me and I abandoned heel cups many years ago. I feel they elevate the heel and put a constant stretch on the plantar fascia (**Fig. 11**).

I also put patients on an NSAID unless they have an absolute contraindication for this class of medication. Another simple modality that I have found helpful is ice. I recommend using a direct ice massage with a water-filled Styrofoam cup that has been frozen and the top half peeled back.

I usually try stretching, NSAIDs, and shoe wear with silicone insoles for 3 weeks. If this is not leading to success, I offer the patient an injection of cortisone early on in treatment. I have injected hundreds of patients for plantar fasciitis and do not have one case of fat atrophy of the heel that I know of. It is important to go directly down to the plantar fascial origin and not inject any of the solution into the fat pad. I do have three cases of plantar fascial rupture that all resolved with immobilization and

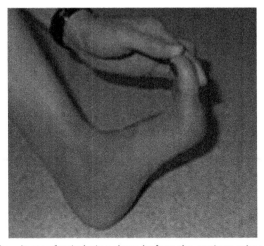

Fig. 9. Stretch of the plantar fascia being done before the patient arises.

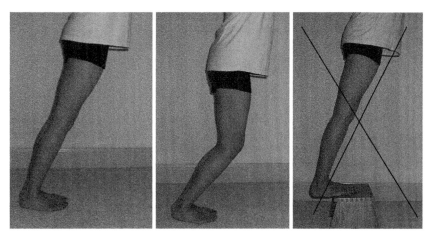

Fig. 10. When patients do an Achilles stretch, I prefer the foot to be flat on the ground. Hanging the heel over a stool or step I have found can make plantar fasciitis worse.

had no long-term problems. I feel it is important to immobilize a rupture of the plantar fascia in a cast or cast boot for a minimum of 4 weeks and then progress to shoes with an orthotic. I always discuss this as a potential complication before injection and discuss how we will manage it if it does happen.

If the patient is having enough symptoms to warrant injection, I also recommend night splints. I tell patients that they are very effective but usually disturb their sleep. Many patients do not tolerate them through the night but most acknowledge benefit if they can wear them. I have found no particular advantage of one type over the other and success depends more on patients being able to tolerate them. I have also found that trying to keep the foot in 5 degrees of dorsiflexion is poorly tolerated and wearing a splint at neutral is still very helpful.

When patients are using an NSAID, silicone insoles, stretching, night splint, and have had an injection, I will stay with the course of treatment and wait a month before I consider a second injection. If they still persist with pain at that time I will do a second injection. At this point, very few patients will remain symptomatic and most are

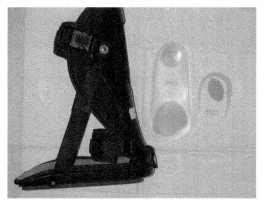

Fig. 11. Three-quarter silicone insole preferred over heel cup.

improved. If patients are still having problems, I will offer them a custom orthotic and have found no one type or fabrication method superior to another. If there is no improvement I will get an MRI scan to be sure I am correct in my diagnosis.

Along with treatment, patients need to modify their lifestyle and avoid activities that have high impact and stretch on the plantar fascia. If the patient is moderately obese, weight loss will help and aerobic activities such as biking, swimming, and an elliptical trainer will be better than treadmills or running.

If you still have a symptomatic patient, continuing with a conservative course of treatment, I feel, is still prudent. I will discuss ESWT but I do not offer this as treatment before 6 months of failure of the previously discussed modalities. I have used both low-energy and high-energy ESWT and feel the high energy may work better but this is only an anecdotal finding. One must remember that this modality may not be covered by insurance.

I do not recommend surgery before a year of treatment, as I find very few patients are not resolved by this time interval. I have no experience with endoscopic plantar fascial release and feel a limited open approach lets me release 50% of the plantar fascia and also release the first branch of the lateral plantar nerve. If there is a heel spur present, I always remove it for fear the patient will fixate on it if he or she still has symptoms after the surgery.

In the truly refractory patient who has had surgery, I am very reluctant to consider another operation. Before considering another operation for the same problem, the clinician first has to consider another diagnosis. Certainly, nerve entrapment is usually high on the list and can be iatrogenic or simply missed at the time of the first operation. This is especially true for an isolated endoscopic release. Unless the diagnosis is very clear, I feel a very conservative approach should be taken in the patient refractory to surgery. In some cases, especially runners, it may be a situation of just more rest being needed.

In summary, plantar fasciitis is a common problem without known etiology. It responds well to multiple conservative modalities and no particular modality has been demonstrated to be clearly superior in the treatment of this condition. Over 90% of patients will be cured by nonoperative treatment but this may require 6 to 12 months of treatment and encouragement by the physician. In the patients who are refractory to the simple conservative modalities, ESWT appears to be the trend. It is noninvasive with a success rate comparable to surgery and has a very low complication rate. Surgery can be done endoscopically or open with very similar long-term outcomes. Patients appear to recover from endoscopic treatment 4 to 5 weeks earlier than the open group. If there is a suggestion of FBLPN entrapment, then patients should have an open release.

REFERENCES

1. Gill LH, Kiebzak GM. Outcome of nonsurgical treatment for plantar fasciitis. Foot Ankle Int 1996;17:527–32.
2. Gill LH. Plantar fasciitis: diagnosis and conservative management. J Am Acad Orthop Surg 1997;5109–17.
3. Tisdel CL. Heel pain, in orthopaedic knowledge update: foot and ankle 3. Rosemont, IL: American Academy of Orthopaedic Surgeons; 2003. p. 113–9.
4. Buchbinder R. Clinical practice: plantar fasciitis. N Engl J Med 2004;350: 2159–66.
5. Graham CE. Painful heel syndrome: rationale of diagnosis and treatment. Foot Ankle 1983;3:261–7.

6. Riddle DL, Schappert SM. Volume of ambulatory care visits and patterns of care for patients diagnosed with plantar fasciitis: a national study of medical doctors. Foot Ankle Int 2004;25:303–31.

7. Davies MS, Weiss GA, Saxby TS. Plantar fasciitis: how successful is surgical intervention? Foot Ankle Int 1999;20:803–7.

8. Saxena A, Fullem B. Plantar fascia ruptures in athletes. Am J Sports Med 2004;32:662–5.

9. Riddle DL, Pulisic M, Pidcoe P, et al. Risk factors for plantar fasciitis: a matched case-control study. J Bone Joint Surg Am 2003;85:872–7.

10. Wolgin M, Cook C, Graham C, et al. Conservative treatment of plantar heel pain: long-term follow-up. Foot Ankle Int 1994;15:97–102.

11. Lapidus PW Guidotti FP. Painful heel: report of 323 patients wth 364 painful heels. Clin Orthop 1965;39:178–86.

12. Myerson M. Foot and ankle disorders. volume 2. W.B Saunders Baltimore MD; 2000.

13. Lee TH. Maurus PB. Plantar heel pain. In: Coughlin MJ, Mann RA, Saltzman CL, editors. Surgery of the foot and ankle. edition 8. vol. 1. Mosby Elsevier Philadelphia; 2007. p. 689–705.

14. Wright DG, Rennels DC. A study of the elastic properties of plantar fascia. J Bone Joint Surg Am 1964;46:482–92.

15. Hicks JH. The mechanics of the foot: II. The plantar aponeurosis and the arch. J Anat 1954;88:25–30.

16. Baxter DE, Pfeffer GB. Treatment of chronic heel pain by surgical release of the first branch of the lateral plantar nerve. Clin Orthop Relat Res 1992;279:229–36.

17. Baxter DE, Thigpen CM. Heel pain: operative results. Foot Ankle 1984;5:16–25.

18. Chang CC, Miltner LJ. Periostitis of the os calcis. J Bone Joint Surg 1934;16:355–64.

19. DuVries HL. Heel spur (calcaneal spur). Arch Surg 1957;74:536–42.

20. Lemont H, Ammirati KM, Usen N. Plantar fasciitis: a degenerative process (fasciosis) without inflammation. J Am Podiatr Med Assoc 2003;93:234–7.

21. Levy JC, Mizel MS, Clifford PD, et al. Value of radiographs in the initial evaluation of nontraumatic adult heel pain. Foot Ankle Int 2006;27:427–30.

22. Williams PL, Smibert JG, Cox R, et al. Imaging study of the painful heel syndrome. Foot Ankle 1987;7:345–9.

23. Akfirat M, Sen C, Gunes T. Ultrasonographic appearance of the plantar fasciitis. Clin Imaging 2003;27:353–7.

24. Kane D, Greaney T, Shanahan M, et al. The role of ultrasonography in the diagnosis and management of idiopathic plantar fasciitis. Rheumatology 2001;40:1002–8.

25. Sabir N, Demirlenk S, Yagci B, et al. Clinical utility of sonography in diagnosing plantar fasciitis. J Ultrasound Med 2005;24:1041–8.

26. Porter D, Barrill E, Oneacre K, et al. The effects of duration and frequency of Achilles tendon stretching on dorsiflexion and outcome in painful heel syndrome. A randomized, blinded, control study. Foot Ankle Int 2002;23(7):619–24.

27. DiGiovanni BF, Nawoczenski DA, Malay DP, et al. Plantar fascia–specific stretching exercise improves outcomes in patients with chronic plantar fasciitis: a prospective clinical trial with two-year follow-up. J Bone Joint Surg Am 2006;88:1775–81.

28. Wapner KL, Sharkey PF. The use of night splints for treatment of recalcitrant plantar fasciitis. Foot Ankle 1991;12:135–7.

29. Powell M, Post WR, Keener J, et al. Effective treatment of chronic plantar fasciitis with dorsiflexion night splints: a crossover prospective randomized outcome study. Foot Ankle Int 1998;19:10–8.

30. Donley BG, Moore T, Sferra J, et al. The efficacy of oral nonsteroidal anti-inflammatory medication (NSAID) in the treatment of plantar fasciitis: a randomized, prospective, placebo-controlled study. Foot Ankle Int 2007;28:20–3.
31. Pfeffer G, Bacchetti P, Deland J, et al. Comparison of custom and prefabricated orthoses in the initial treatment of proximal plantar fasciitis. Foot Ankle Int 1999; 20:214–21.
32. Landorf KB, Keenan A, Herbert RD. Effectiveness of foot orthoses to treat plantar fasciitis: a randomized trial. Arch Intern Med 2006;166:1305–10.
33. Crawford F, Atkins D, Young P, et al. Steroid injections for heel pain: evidence of short-term effectiveness. A randomized controlled trial. Rheumatology 1999;38:974–7.
34. Miller RA, Torres J, Mcguire M. Efficacy of first-time steroid injections for painful heel syndrome. Foot Ankle Int 1995;16(16):610–2.
35. Acevedo JI, Beskin JL. Complications of plantar fascia rupture associated with corticosteroid injection. Foot Ankle Int 1998;19:91–7.
36. Sellman JR. Plantar fascia rupture associated with corticosteroid injection. Foot Ankle Int 1994;15(7):376–81.
37. Babcock MS, Foster L, Pasquina P, et al. Treatment of pain attributed to plantar fasciitis with botulinum toxin A: a short-term, randomized, placebo-controlled, double-blind study. Am J Phys Med Rehabil 2005;84:649–54.
38. Placzek R, Deuretzbacher G, Meiss AL, et al. Treatment of chronic plantar fasciitis with botulinum toxin A. Clin J Pain 2006;22:190–2.
39. Hlavac HF. The Foot Book: Advice for Athletes. Mountain View, CA: World Publications, Inc.
40. Scranton PE, Pedegana LR, Whitesel JP. Gait analysis. Alterations in support phase forces using supportive devices. AM J Sports Med 1982;10(1):6–11.
41. Radford JA , Landorf KB, Buchbinder R, et al. Effectiveness of low-Dye taping for the short-term treatment of plantar heel pain: a randomized trial. BMC Musculoskeletal Disorders 2006. Available at: http://www.biomedcentral.com/logon/logon. asp?msg=ce>.
42. Tisdel CL, Harper MC. Chronic plantar heel pain: treatment with a short leg walking cast. Foot Ankle Int 1996;17:41–2.
43. Chen HS, Chen LM, Huang TW. Treatment of painful heel syndrome with shock waves. Clin Orthop Relat Res 2001;387:41–6.
44. Maier M, Steinborn M, Schmitz C, et al. Extracorporeal shock wave application for chronic plantar fasciitis associated with heel spurs: prediction of outcome by magnetic resonance imaging. J Rheumatol 2000;27:2455–62.
45. Rompe JD, Decking J, Schoellner C, et al. Shock wave application for chronic plantar fasciitis in running athletes: a prospective, randomized, placebo-controlled trial. Am J Sports Med 2003;31:268–75.
46. Buch M, Knorr U, Fleming L, et al. Extracorporeal shockwave therapy in symptomatic heel spurs: An overview. Orthopade 2002;31:637–44.
47. Kudo P, Dainty K, Clarfield M, et al. Randomized, placebo-controlled, double-blind clinical trial evaluating the treatment of plantar fasciitis with an extracorporeal shockwave therapy (ESWT) device: a North American confirmatory study. J Orthop Res 2006;24:115–23.
48. Wang CJ, Wang FS, Yang KD, et al. Long-term results of extracorporeal shock-wave treatment for plantar fasciitis. Am J Sports Med 2006;34:592–6.
49. Ogden JA, Alvarez R, Levitt R, et al. Shock wave therapy for chronic proximal plantar fasciitis. Clin Orthop Relat Res 2001;387:47–59.
50. Leach RE, Seavey MS, Salter DK. Results of surgery in athletes with plantar fasciitis. Foot Ankle 1986;7:156–61.

51. Watson TS, Anderson RB, Davis WH, et al. Distal tarsal tunnel release with partial plantar fasciotomy for chronic heel pain: an outcome analysis. Foot Ankle Int 2002;23(6):530–7.
52. Sammarco GJ, Helfrey RB. Surgical treatment of recalcitrant plantar fasciitis. Foot Ankle Int 1996;17(9):520–6.
53. Conflitti JM, Tarquinio TA. Operative outcome of partial plantar fasciectomy and neurolysis to the nerve of the abductor digiti minimi muscle for recalcitrant plantar fasciitis. Foot Ankle Int 2004;25:482–7.
54. Manoli A, Harper MC 2nd, Fitzgibbons TC, et al. Calcaneal fracture after cortical bone removal. Foot Ankle 1992;13(9):523–5.
55. Kinley S, Frascone S, Calderone D, et al. Endoscopic plantar fasciotomy versus traditional heel spur surgery: a prospective study. J Foot Ankle Surg 1993;32(6): 595–603.
56. Brekke MK, Green DR. Retrospective analysis of minimal-incision, endoscopic, and open procedures for heel spur syndrome. J Am Podiatr Med Assoc 1998; 88(2):64–72.
57. Sharkey NA, Donohue SW, Ferris L. Biomechanical consequences of plantar fascial release or rupture during gait. Part II. Alterations in forefoot loading. Foot Ankle Int 1999;29(2):86–96.
58. Thordarson DB, Kumar PJ, Hedman TP, et al. Effect of partial versus complete fasciotomy on the windless mechanism. Foot Ankle Int 1997;18(1):16–20.
59. Daly PJ, Kitaoka HB, Chao EY. Plantar fasciotomy for intractable plantar fasciitis: clinical results and biomechanical evaluation. Foot Ankle 1992;13(4):188–95.
60. Gormley J, Kuwada GT. Retrospective analysis of calcaneal spur removal and complete plantar fascial release for the treatment of chronic heel pain. J Foot Surg 1992;31(2):166–9.
61. Crawford F, Thomson C. Interventions for treating plantar heel pain. Cochrane Database Syst Rev 2003;3:CD000416.
62. Sever JW. Apophysistis of the os calcis. NY Med 1912;95:1025–9.
63. Ferguson AB, Gingrich RM. The abnormal calcaneal apophysis and tarsal navicular. Clin Orthop 1957;10:87–95.
64. Scharfbillig RW, Jones S, Scutter SD. Sever's Disease: What Does the Literature Really Tell Us? J Am Podiatr Med Assoc 2008;98(3):212–23.

Achilles Tendon Ruptures, Re Rupture with Revision Surgery, Tendinosis, and Insertional Disease

Mark A. Krahe, DO[a],*, Gregory C. Berlet, MD[a,b]

KEYWORDS

• Achilles tendinopathy • Tendinosis • Repair • Re-rupture

Achilles tendon pathology is one of the more common conditions encountered by the foot and ankle surgeon. While it most frequently affects the athletic population, it can also lead to significant morbidity in the older and sedentary patient. The etiology of Achilles tendon dysfunction is multifactorial and has been found to be associated with overuse injury, training error, malalignment of the lower extremity, inflammatory disorders, and intrinsic disease or degeneration. Achilles tendon disorders have been classified temporally as acute and chronic, with the later subdivided into insertional and noninsertional (intrinsic) involvement. Histopathology has contributed a great deal to the understanding of disease process. Classification systems have been developed in an attempt to determine methods of treatment and prognosis. This article reviews the clinical spectrum of disease and presents contemporary treatment options.

ANATOMY

The Achilles tendon complex or triceps surae comprises the two heads of the gastrocnemius joining the soleus 12 to 15 cm proximal to the calcaneus. The complex rotates approximately 90° before its broad insertion into the middle of the posterior calcaneal tuberosity. During its contraction, the tendon performs a wringing motion, which, according to hypothesis, creates relative hypoxia. The tendon, lacking a true synovial sheath, is lined by a paratenon with both visceral and parietal layers. The paratenon

[a] Department of Orthopedics, Orthopedic Foot & Ankle Center, 300 Polaris Parkway, Suite 2000, Westerville, OH 43082
[b] Division of Foot and Ankle, Department of Orthopedics, Orthopedic Foot & Ankle Center, Ohio State University, 300 Polaris Parkway, Suite 2000, Westerville, OH 43082, USA
* Corresponding author.
E-mail address: markakrahe@hotmail.com (M.A. Krahe).

Foot Ankle Clin N Am 14 (2009) 247–275
doi:10.1016/j.fcl.2009.04.003
1083-7515/09/$ – see front matter © 2009 Elsevier Inc. All rights reserved.

foot.theclinics.com

comprises mucopolysaccharides that promote tendon glide, allowing for nearly 1.5 cm of excursion.[1,2]

The blood supply to the Achilles is predominantly through the paratenon. The mesotenon contains a series of traversing vincula through which blood vessels can reach the tendon.[3,4] Other sources of vascularity include the musculotendinous junction of the gastrocsoleus complex and the osseous insertion into the calcaneus. Vascular studies have identified a watershed area roughly 2 to 6 cm proximal to the Achilles insertion into the calcaneus. This relatively devascularized area is the most common site for acute tears.

ACUTE ACHILLES RUPTURES

The Achilles tendon is one of the most commonly ruptured tendons in the human body.[5] Bhandari[6] reported an annual incidence of 18 ruptures per 100,000 people. The injuries typically occur in males between the ages of 30 to 50 years, and account for approximately 40% of all operative tendon repairs.[7] The male-to-female ratio reported by Carden and colleagues[8] ranges from 2:1 to 19:1.

Evaluation

The diagnosis of an Achilles tendon tear is typically established by a thorough history and physical examination. Common symptoms of an acute tendon rupture include the feeling of being kicked or shot above the heel following a traumatic event. Patients typically present with marked ambulatory dysfunction, swelling, and palpable gap indicative of a full-thickness tear.

Those with an attritional tear may present with increased swelling or ambulatory dysfunction without a history of trauma. They often do not complain of severe pain, which often accompanies an acute rupture. According to Inglis and Sculco,[9] Achilles tendon ruptures may go undiagnosed by the primary treating physician in up to 23% of cases. Hansen[10] noted that ruptures can often be missed because of diffuse swelling that may mimic a common ankle sprain, especially if the patient delays initial examination by a few days and keeps the ankle in a dependent position.[11] Some patients may be able to perform a single heel rise but generally cannot do so repetitively. Patients may also present with increased ankle dorsiflexion.

Malalignment of the lower extremity is commonly found in patients presenting with Achilles injury. Excess pronation, along with the associated conditions of flat foot, decreased subtalar motion, equinus contracture, and genu varum, are the most common contributing abnormalities. The equinus contracture, which influences the posture of the foot, is the most likely link between these conditions. Conditions related to shock absorption, such as cavus foot and muscle fatigue, have also been associated with Achilles tears.

Imaging

Radiographs are not diagnostic for an Achilles tendon rupture but may demonstrate additional pathology and provide information on the overall alignment of the foot and ankle. When possible, weight-bearing anteroposterior, lateral, and oblique/mortise views of both the foot and ankle should be obtained. Radiographs commonly demonstrate calcification within the tendon, cortical erosions, enthesmophytes, or a Haglund deformity. They can also rule out a calcaneal tuberosity avulsion fracture. Ultrasonography and MRI are performed to confirm diagnosis and determine the extent of tendon retraction. Ultrasound has the advantage of dynamic examination and is more cost-effective than MRI. However, ultrasound is user- and reader-dependent. MRI, on the other hand, allows for the identification of the various stages of disease as well as concomitant pathology. It allows for multiplanar imaging and can be useful in planning surgical reconstruction. MRI and ultrasound are often not needed to make the diagnosis in the routine setting, with a typical history and lack of plantarflexion with the Thompson test.

Pathophysiology

The prologue of Achilles tendon pathology before a complete tear is open to debate. Most investigators would agree that it is a multifactorial process. Studies have shown that more than 75% of ruptures occur during sports-related activities, and chronic painful conditions are common among middle-aged recreational athletes.[12] It is hypothesized that there is an association with overuse from repetitive loading but there has been no direct correlation with physical activity and histopathology.[13] Without a direct correlation of activity to disease, attention has focused on anatomic cohorts associated with Achilles symptoms.

The most common location for Achilles rupture is the watershed area approximately 2 to 6 cm proximal to the insertion. It is theorized that tears occur in this region secondary to high mechanical stress and relative hypovascularity. Tendons behave viscoelastically and exhibit adaptive responses to conditions of increased loading and disuse.[2] Ultimate tendon stress leads to failure, resulting in either partial or complete tear.

Immediately following a tear, hematomas form secondary to vascular insult. The aggregation of platelets releases proinflammatory mediators, recruiting leukocytes, neutrophils, and macrophages, inducing the formation of extracellular matrix, fibroblast proliferation, and removal of necrotic tissue.[14] The injured cells are responsible for the release of and response to local factors, leading to collagen production and repair.

Following an acute tendon rupture, interposed hematoma or lack of prompt immobilization in plantarflexion can result in loss of tendon apposition leading to scar formation, healing in a lengthened position, or both. Ideally, early immobilization with tendon apposition allows for maintenance of tendon length and remodeling potential for "tendon" healing (**Fig. 1**).

MANAGEMENT OF ACUTE ACHILLES TEARS

Controversy surrounds the choice of operative versus nonoperative treatment of acute Achilles tendon tears. Common goals to both options include restoration of tendon

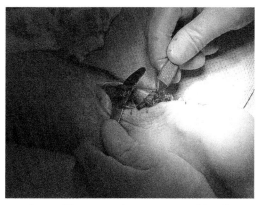

Fig. 1. Acute Achilles rupture with mop-end appearance of tendinous ends. The plantaris tendon remains intact.

length, tension, and function. Ideally the patient would be able to return to their pre-morbid activity level. Most investigators would agree that refinement of the surgical technique has led to lower complication rates, making surgical treatment the preferred method for younger patients and competitive athletes, as well as for the active elderly population. Nonoperative treatment remains the standard for those with multiple medical comorbidities and those at high risk for wound complications.

Advocates for nonoperative treatment of Achilles ruptures report a decreased complication rate of wound infections, skin necrosis, and nerve injury. Nonoperative treatment of an Achilles rupture requires the foot to be placed into an equinus position resulting in approximation of the tendon ends to promote "end-to-end" healing. This can be achieved in either a cast or boot. Patients are typically immobilized for 6 to 8 weeks before initiating range-of-motion exercises. Ultrasound must be performed within the first couple weeks of treatment to confirm apposition of the tendon ends. Residual diastasis is a relative indication to switch to surgical treatment.

Complications following nonoperative treatment of an Achilles rupture may result in lengthening of the tendon, which alters mechanics and decreases push-off strength. Silver and colleagues[15–17] reported a 10% to 35% rerupture rate with nonsurgical treatment and immobilization in a plaster cast. Certainly ambulatory dysfunction secondary to weakness and gait disturbance can have a significant impact on morbidity and mortality in the elderly population. There is also a significant productivity and financial burden for those who rerupture or fail nonoperative treatment.

The most common postoperative complications after acute repair include infection and delayed wound-healing. Other general complications of Achilles surgery include rerupture, healing in a lengthened position (incorrect tensioning), deep venous thrombosis, pulmonary embolus, and peritendinous calcification or scar.

Superficial postoperative infections usually respond to a course of oral antibiotics. When there is evidence of deep infection, hospitalization with a course of intravenous antibiotics and return to the operating suite for irrigation and debridement may be warranted. Infected cavitary skin and soft tissue defects can be treated with a wound vacuum system allowing for local wound debridement and healing by secondary intention. If a large skin defect remains in the absence of infection, then a full-thickness skin graft may be used.

Hufner and colleagues[18] studied the long-term results of functional nonoperative treatment of acute Achilles tendon ruptures in a high-shaft boot with a 3-cm hindfoot elevation. The indications for treatment in the boot included a distance of 10 mm or less between the tendon ends with the ankle in neutral and complete apposition at 20° plantarflexion confirmed by ultrasound. One hundred and twenty-five patients were followed for a mean of 5.5 years from injury. Subjective and objective outcome measures included good or excellent outcome in 92 (73.5%) patients with complete rehabilitation and return to sport at preinjury level. Satisfactory (9%) and poor results (17.5%) were due to pain in the Achilles, lengthened tendon, reduced strength, and marked reduction in calf size. Eight patients developed rerupture (8.7%).

Bhandari and colleagues[6] performed a meta-analysis of randomized trials for acute Achilles ruptures (five studies, 336 patients). They found a statistically significant reduced risk of rerupture when comparing open repair versus conservative treatment for acute tears (3.6% versus 10.6% rerupture). Infection rates from open repairs varied from 4% to 20%. The relative risk of infection with surgical repair was 5.2 times greater than that for cast treatment.

Cetti and colleagues[7] reported on a prospective randomized series of 111 patients with acute Achilles tears treated with either operative or nonoperative treatment. They noted a 4% deep-infection rate in the operative group and a 13% rerupture rate in the nonoperative group. Fifty-seven percent of patients treated operatively were able to return to work and sport without restrictions, while only 29% in the nonoperative group met this goal.

Khan and colleagues[19] performed a meta-analysis of randomized controlled trials for operative and nonoperative treatment of acute Achilles tendon ruptures. A scoring system was established for methodology, and 12 of 36 published studies met criteria for inclusion. A total of 800 people participated. The study concluded that open operative treatment was associated with a lower risk of rerupture compared with nonoperative treatment, 3.5% versus 12.6%. However, operative treatment was associated with a higher risk of infections, adhesions, and disturbed skin sensibility. The pooled rate of reported complications for the operative group (other than rerupture) was 34.1% compared with 2.7% in the nonoperative group. When comparing open repair versus percutaneous, the open group had a rerupture rate of 4.3%, while the rate for the percutaneous group was 2.1%. The rate of complications excluding rerupture for open group was 26.1% and 8.3% for percutaneous repair. The open group had an infection rate of 19.6% while that for the percutaneous group was 0%. In comparing postoperative cast immobilization alone with cast immobilization followed by functional bracing, rerupture rates were 5.0% in the cast immobilization group and 2.3% in the functional bracing group. Complications were the highest in the cast-only group for adhesions (18.6% compared with 9.7% in cast followed by bracing), disturbed sensibility (8.6% compared with 9.7%), keloid or hypertrophic scarring (5% versus 3%), and infection (3.5% compared with 3%).

SURGICAL TREATMENT FOR ACUTE ACHILLES RUPTURE

Direct end-to-end anastamosis can usually be performed following an acute rupture. It is important to allow for swelling to subside before surgery. The soft tissue envelope must be respected to prevent any postoperative healing complications. A medial approach is typically performed to prevent iatrogenic injury to the sural nerve. The same incision can also be later used for revision surgery with flexor hallucis longus (FHL) tendon transfer. Dissection is carried down to the paratenon, which is incised longitudinally and reflected to expose the tendon ends. A posterior compartment fasciotomy as described by Mandelbaum and Myerson[20] can be performed to effectively increase the volume of the posterior compartment, allowing for decreased tension on the repair. The mop ends of the tear are then freshened to facilitate reapproximation. Biomechanically, the Krackow suture technique using a nonstrangulating locking stitch has been shown to be stronger than the Bunnell or modified Kessler stitch.[21] Load to failure using two core strands of suture shows 147 N for the Krackow stitch, 93 N for the Bunnel stitch, and 85 N for the modified Kessler stitch.[22,23] Once excursion of the proximal tendon is achieved, the suture limbs are tensioned and tied. There should not be a gap in the repair. The opposite extremity can also be used to ensure appropriate tensioning. The paratenon is then repaired over the tendon to facilitate healing. Standard layered closure is then performed (**Fig. 2**).

Clinicians can choose from a variety of rehabilitation protocols following open surgical repair of an acute Achilles tendon rupture. Treatment options vary from complete immobilization with casting to immediate weight-bearing. There is no consensus as to which technique is superior. Suchak and colleagues[24–26] performed a level-one study comparing early weight-bearing verse non–weight-bearing following surgical repair of an acute Achilles tendon rupture. Ninety-eight patients completed a 6-month follow-up. At 6 weeks, the weight-bearing group had significantly better scores than the non–weight-bearing group in the Rand-36 domains of physical

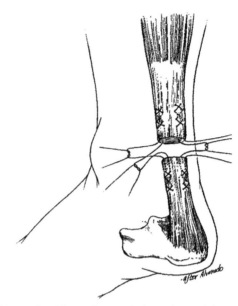

Fig. 2. Primary Achilles repair with Krackow technique. (*From* Saltzman C, Tearse D. Achilles tendon injuries. J Am Acad Orthop Surg 1998;6(5):323. Copyright © 1998 American Academy of Orthopedic Surgeons.)

functioning, social functioning, role-emotional, and vitality scores ($P<.05$). Patients in the weight-bearing group also reported fewer limitations of daily activities at 6 weeks postoperatively ($P<.001$). At 6 months, there was no significant difference between the groups. Both groups demonstrated poor endurance of the calf musculature, and no one in either group developed a rerupture. The study concluded that early weight-bearing following acute Achilles tendon repair improves health-related quality of life in the early postoperative period and has no detrimental effect on recovery.

PERCUTANEOUS REPAIR

In 1977, Ma and Griffith[27,28] introduced the idea of a limited open or percutaneous repair of an acute Achilles tendon rupture. This technique involves making small vertical incisions along the medial and lateral border of the Achilles tendon. The incisions facilitate the passage of suture through the rupture tendon ends and allow for anastomosis. The goal was to reduce postoperative wound complications, allow visualization of the tendon stumps for accurate reapproximation, and facilitate early rehabilitation (**Fig. 3**).

Hockenbury and Johns[29,30] compared in vitro percutaneous repair of the Achilles with open repair using transverse tenotomy in 10 fresh-frozen cadavers. The open repair group used the Bunnell suture technique and the percutaneous group used the classic Ma and Griffith procedure.[27] The open technique resisted nearly twice the amount of ankle dorsiflexion before a 10-mm gap was obtained (27.6° compared with 14.4°). Entrapment of the sural nerve occurred in 3 of the 5 specimens that had a percutaneous repair. Investigators also noted that 4 of 5 specimens examined after percutaneous repair demonstrated malalignment.

To date, few prospective randomized studies have compared percutaneous/mini-open techniques with open Achilles repair. Lim and colleagues[31,32] studied 33 patients

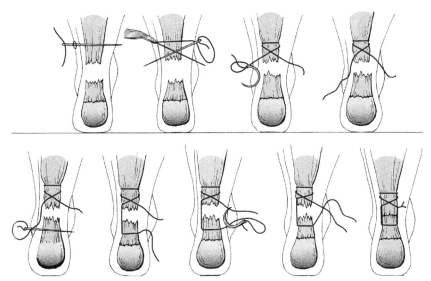

Fig. 3. Ma and Griffith technique. (*From* Coughlin M, Mann R, Saltzman C. Surgery of the foot and ankle. 8th edition. Philadelphia: Mosby; 2007. p. 1245; with permission.)

randomized to a modified Ma and Griffith percutaneous technique compared with 33 patients getting a standard open repair with Kessler suture technique. Mean age was 38.5 years. Forty patients were male and 26 female. The mean duration of immobilization was 12.4 weeks. Complications in the open group included seven wound infections (21%), two adhesions (6%), and two cases of rerupture (6%). In the percutaneous group, there were three cases of wound puckering (9%), one rerupture (3%), and one case with persistent paresthesia in the sural nerve distribution (3%). The difference in infective wound complications between the two groups was statistically significant in favor of percutaneous repair.

Assal and colleagues[33,34] reported on a cadaveric study to develop the Achillon instrumentation system for percutaneous repair of acute Achilles tendon ruptures. They reported on a consecutive series of 83 patients treated with the device at three level-one Swiss hospitals. Postoperative American Orthopaedic Foot and Ankle Scores (AOFAS) at 26-month follow-up was a mean of 96 points. Isokinetic and endurance testing revealed no significant difference compared with the uninjured side. No sural nerve injuries were documented.

Most studies reporting on athletes with an Achilles repair have involved the middle-aged recreational athlete. The early motion and early weight-bearing approaches after an open repair have been effective. With an aggressive rehabilitation approach, return to sports can be between 6 to 12 months. Professional athletes can typically return the next season after a repair.

CHRONIC ACHILLES RUPTURE/RERUPTURE

The definition of an old, chronic, or neglected rupture is debatable. Clancy and colleagues[35] developed a classification system based upon the duration of rupture. Acute ruptures are denoted as those less than 2 weeks old. Subacute injuries are from 3 to 6 weeks old, while chronic disease is anything exceeding 6 weeks.

The chronic disease process entails disorganized scar tissue that fills the gap between the retracted stumps. The fibrous tissue lacks any significant orientation, resulting in weakness and marked adhesions. As early as 1956, Bosworth[36] noted that contraction of the tendon ends typically occurs within 3 to 4 days following an acute rupture. This set the precedence as to why acute ruptures treated by nonoperative intervention require immobilization in plantar-flexion within 48 hours from injury.

Evaluation

Examination should include all of the components previously discussed for a suspected acute rupture. Because of the incorporation of fibrous tissue, the athlete may not have a palpable gap between the rupture tendon ends. Plantarflexion strength should be assessed closely. Athletes may compensate by recruiting the posterior tibialis tendon and FHL tendon to aid in plantarflexion. Active plantarflexion, however, should be weaker than the contralateral extremity in lieu of the injured tendon.

Delayed presentation, chronic Achilles rupture, or rerupture can make reconstruction difficult. In a situation where there is retraction or tendon loss, end-to-end anastomosis may not be achievable and surgical treatment can require augmentation.[37,38] Various treatment modalities have been described, such as turn-down flaps, allografts, local tendon transfers, and even synthetic augmentation. Successful reconstruction must include tendon repair or transfer sufficient to provide strength, durability, and tension for athletic performance.

When planning revision surgery, soft tissue coverage must be thick enough to withstand repetitive friction and the shearing forces encountered during ambulation. Also, the coverage must allow for comfortable shoe wear.[39] Clinicians should be mindful of previous incisions to prevent skin necrosis. When clinical examination demonstrates vascular compromise, appropriate vascular consultation should be performed before surgery. The surgeon must try to identify the cause of failure. Complex revision surgery should be avoided when a patient has demonstrated postoperative noncompliance leading to failure. Infectious etiology should be ruled out also. If planning a tendon transfer, the patient must demonstrate a minimum 4 out of 5 strength from the donor tendon without spasticity. Alternative procedures should be planned for patients that previously demonstrated a hypersensitivity reaction to allograft or xenograft soft tissue augments (**Fig. 4**).

SURGICAL OPTIONS FOR CHRONIC ACHILLES RUPTURE/RERUPTURE

Christensen in 1931[40] was the first to report surgical treatment of neglected Achilles tendon ruptures. He described a turn-down flap technique to bridge the tendon gap. A distally based 2-cm by 10-cm flap was cut in the proximal tendon fragment, then turned down to cover the tendon defect or previous repair. Postoperatively, the patients were placed in an above-the-knee equinus cast for 5 weeks followed by a walking below-the-knee cast for 5 weeks. In a reported series of 35 tears, he noted 2 reruptures and 75% "satisfactory" outcome. One of the disadvantages of this repair includes the development of a large tissue mass that can occasionally be irritating to the patient. This may delay or lead to wound complications secondary to excessive tension to the overlying skin. Turn-down flaps tend to be limited in width and length and are therefore more of an augmentation than a replacement.

In 1975, Abraham and Pankovich[41] described a tendo-Achilles advancement with an inverted V incision at the musculotendinous junction. The arms of the V were at least 1.5 times the length of the tendon defect to allow suturing of the incision in a Y configuration. They determined that gaps up to 6 cm could be closed with this

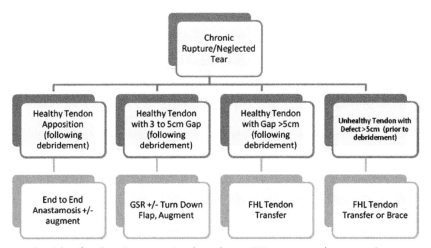

Fig. 4. Algorithm for chronic rupture/neglected tear. GSR, gastroc-soleus recession.

technique. They had a limited series of four patients documented and reported that three patients gained full strength of the Achilles and one had "slight weakness." There was one documented complication of a sural neuroma (**Fig. 5**).

Tendon Transfers for Chronic Achilles Ruptures/Reruptures

The goal of tendon transfer is to replicate the tension and line of pull of the defective tendon without providing any additional functional morbidity. In an attempt to refine surgical techniques, Silver and colleagues[15] described the relative strength percentages of the muscles surrounding the foot and ankle. Collectively, the plantar flexors represent 54.5% of the total strength. The gastrocsoleus complex generates

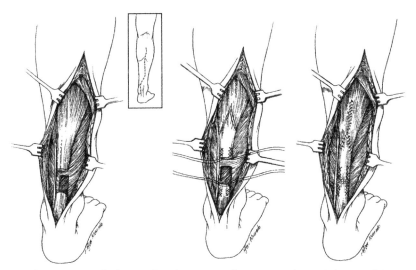

Fig. 5. Defect is spanned after performing a V-Y advancement.(*From* Saltzman C, Tearse D. Achilles tendon injuries. J Am Acad Orthop Surg 1998;6(5):324; with permission. Copyright © 1998 American Academy of Orthopedic Surgeons.)

49.1%. The FHL, being the second strongest plantar-flexor, contributes 3.6%. The flexor digitorum longus (FDL) provides 1.8% and the peroneus brevis provides 2.6%.

Roger Mann[42] introduced the idea of using an FDL tendon transfer for a chronic Achilles rupture. He reported on a series of seven patients treated with a two-incision technique. A medial incision was used to release the FDL distal to the knot of Henry. A second posteromedial incision was used to tunnel the FDL through the calcaneus and suture to itself. This was performed in conjunction with a gastrocnemius turn-down flap. The average follow-up was 39 months. Two patients required an adjuvant procedure (rotational flap and skin graft). No reruptures occurred. Six patients reported good results. One reported a fair result.

Another option for chronic rupture or rerupture includes the FHL tendon transfer. Measuring an average of 8 to 10 cm long and 4 to 5 mm wide, the FHL tendon allows for sufficient augmentation of the Achilles tendon.[43,44] The long, distal reaching muscle belly of the FHL brings well-vascularized tissue to the critical area of the Achilles, which is relatively avascular (typically 2 to 6 cm proximal to the calcaneal insertion). The FHL is the second strongest plantar flexor of the ankle with its axis of contractile force most closely aligned to the Achilles tendon. Its neuromuscular activation, in phase with the triceps surae muscle, supports a normal gait cycle. In comparison to other tendon options, the FHL has anatomic proximity to the Achilles, thus allowing for relatively straightforward dissection with less risk of iatrogenic injury to the neurovascular bundle (**Fig. 6**).

Since Hansen first described the FHL tendon transfer for the augmentation of Achilles tendon defects, numerous modifications have been introduced. Wapner

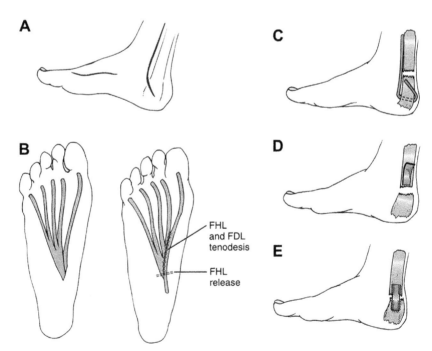

Fig. 6. FHL tendon transfer. Two-incision technique as originally described by Hansen. (*From* Coughlin M, Mann R, Saltzman C. Surgery of the foot and ankle. 8th edition. Philadelphia: Mosby; 2007. p. 1234; with permission.)

and colleagues[45] performed a prospective study of eight patients treated for chronic Achilles tendon rupture with a FHL tendon transfer. The average follow-up was 17 months with a mean age of 52 years. The outcomes measured included postoperative range of motion, scar healing, sensation, motor strength with Cybex testing, and patient satisfaction based upon a questionnaire.

The surgical technique used two incisions, one on the medial border of the midfoot with release of the distal FHL and the other a posteromedial incision to expose the Achilles and its insertion into the calcaneus. Once the FHL was released, it was tunneled through the Achilles and woven into the Achilles to bridge the gap. The plantaris tendon was also woven into the repair for additional strength.

Three patients had no pain postoperatively without any limitations and excellent strength. Three patients had good result, meaning at least neutral dorsiflexion, no postoperative wound complications, and return to preoperative occupation and athletic activity. One person had a fair result with significant weakness in all muscle groups of the ankle.

There were no poor results and no reruptures were documented. All patients had some minor loss of passive range of motion to flexion of the great toe interphalangeal joint, but none of the patients had noticed this on follow-up examination until it was brought up in conversation. Cybex testing at 30° per second noted an average decrease of 29.5% in plantarflexion power compared with the normal contralateral extremity. Additionally, no patients developed a hammer-toe deformity.

Pearsall and colleagues[46] described a two-incision technique for Achilles tendon repair similar to Wapner with the modification of interference screw fixation if the FHL was too short to route through the calcaneus and suture to itself.

Decarbo and Hyer[47–49] described another FHL tendon transfer technique using a short harvest. This technique involved a single posteromedial incision with a short FHL harvest and transfer to the calcaneus tuberosity with interference screw fixation (**Figs. 7–16**). **Figs. 9–14** demonstrate the steps of this short-harvest technique.

Cottom and colleagues[50] reported on the largest series of patients treated with the short FHL tendon transfer method (as described by Decarbo and Hyer). Sixty-two patients with chronic Achilles tendinopathy underwent debridement and transfer of the FHL tendon when greater than 50% of the tendon was involved. All 62 patients were followed for an average of 26.9 months. Outcomes measured included the modified AOFAS both preoperatively and postoperatively.

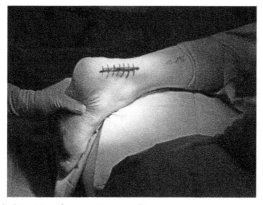

Fig. 7. Planned medial incision for excising tendinosis.

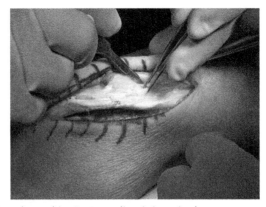

Fig. 8. After incision planned in **Fig. 7**, tendinosis is excised.

Achilles tendons were evaluated by MRI before surgery. Severely damaged tendons required excision. A preoperative and postoperative modified AOFAS system demonstrated significant improvement after surgery (average preoperative modified hindfoot AOFAS was 20.4; average postoperative hindfoot AOFAS was 51.5). Nine cases of superficial cellulitis and five cases of minor wound dehiscence were noted.

Hahn and colleagues[43] performed a study to evaluate postoperative MRI based on clinical outcome and isokinetic strength in 13 patients with chronic Achilles tendinopathy who underwent augmentation with FHL transfer. Clinical parameters as well as AOFAS and SF-36 scoring were reported after an average follow-up of 46.5 months. Qualitative analyses and MRI of the operative and nonoperative side were compared. Investigators noted that all patients had a significant reduction of pain following surgery. The operated side had a torque deficit of 35% for plantar flexion. Ten patients returned to their former level of activity. MRI showed a complete integration of the FHL tendon is 6 patients. Fatty atrophy of the Achilles was noted in 10 patients. The FHL was free of degeneration in all patients. In fact, hypertrophy was noted of the FHL in 8 patients. The study concluded that FHL transfer is a valuable treatment option for chronic Achilles tendinopathy both with and without rupture. Results show high patient satisfaction without donor-site morbidity. The FHL tendon is well integrated in the repair. The primary benefit of this procedure was pain relief as well as increased muscle strength.

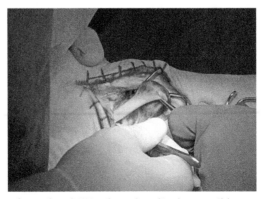

Fig. 9. Fasciotomy performed and FHL released as distal as possible.

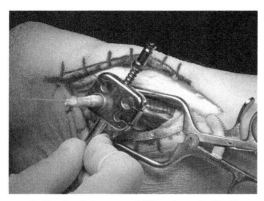

Fig. 10. Tendon measured after fasciotomy and FHL release in **Fig. 9**.

Soft Tissue Augments

A number of soft tissue augments are currently on the market. Allograft and xenograft options are both available. Regardless of what type of soft tissue scaffold is used, soft tissue augments are to be strictly used as an adjuvant, and should never be used to span a defect.

The GraftJacket Regenerative Tissue Matrix (Wright Medical Technology, Arlington, Tennessee) is a scaffold material processed from donated human skin supplied from United States tissue banks. The allograft skin is processed to remove both epidermal and dermal cells while preserving the remaining bioactive components and structure of dermis. This allows for a framework to support cellular repopulation and vascular in-growth. This allograft skin has the potential for incorporation as well as remodeling.

As with any allograft, there is the possibility of disease transmission. Careful donor screening as well as testing for hepatitis B and C, HIV, human T-lymphotrophic virus, bacterial/fungal pathogens, and syphilis are performed under the Food and Drug Administration or Centers for Disease Control and Prevention recommendations. Despite all measures, existing tests cannot provide absolute assurance that the graft will not transmit disease. Other potential complications of the graft material include hypersensitivity reaction, resorption of the matrix, and nonintegration with the host tissue.

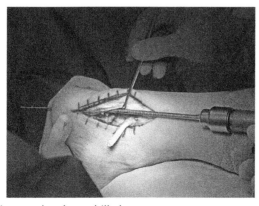

Fig. 11. Steinman pin passed and overdrilled.

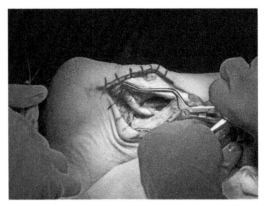

Fig. 12. Suture is passed through tunnel to plantar aspect of foot, then tensioned.

After rehydration, the graft is soft and pliable, allowing for it to be manipulated and conformed to the repair. It can be used as an intercalary support or tubularized around a repair to provide additional strength (**Figs. 17–19**).

A xenograft tissue scaffold is another option for augmenting a repair. The products differ by the source with scaffold from bovine, porcine, and equine sources all currently available. Similar to their allograft counterpart, they provide an acellular organized collagen scaffold that allows ingrowth and remodeling of normal tendon or ligament. They do not have the associated risk of HIV or hepatitis transmission, but there have been documented cases of inflammatory reactions (**Figs. 20–22**).

STAGES OF ACHILLES INFLAMMATION AND DEGENERATION

Clain and Baxter[12] separated Achilles tendon dysfunction into insertional and noninsertional tendinitis. Insertional tendinitis occurs within or around the tendon at the calcaneal insertion. Noninsertional tendinitis occurs in proximity to the insertion. The term tendinitis has since been modified because histologic analysis has shown that the Achilles lacks a true synovial sheath and has a paucity of intrinsic vascularity, making it relatively resistant to inflammation. This has led to the development of

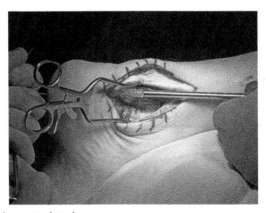

Fig. 13. Biotenodesis screw placed.

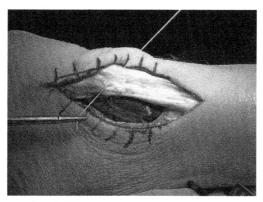

Fig. 14. FHL fascia sutured to Achilles.

a standard classification system guiding treatment. Puddu and colleagues[51] proposed the three stages of Achilles inflammation and degeneration: paratenonitis, tendinosis, and paratenonitis with tendinosis.

Paratenonitis

Paratenonitis is an inflammatory process of the paratenon and surrounding tissue. In most cases, the paratenon is thickened and adherent to the tendon. Histologic analysis reveals fibrous exudates within the diseased Achilles paratenon.

Physical examination findings consistent with paratenonitis include increased warmth and tenderness with a palpable nonmobile area of thickening or induration. Crepitance may be detected while taking the Achilles through range of motion.

Initial treatment includes activity modification, rest, and immobilization. The inflammatory changes of paratenonitis may respond to nonsteroidal anti-inflammatory medications and icing. A brisement technique where the pseudosheath of the paratenon is injected with a local anesthetic under image guidance followed by mobilization can break up adhesions and improve function.

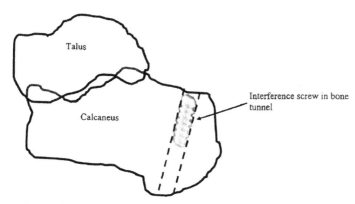

Fig. 15. Lateral view showing appropriate placement of biotenodesis screw. (*From* Decarbo WT, Hyer CF. Interference screw fixation for flexor hallucis longus tendon transfer for chronic Achilles tendonopathy. J Foot Ankle Surg 2008;47(1):71; with permission.)

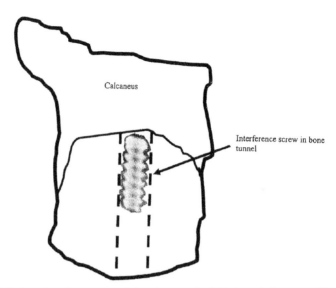

Fig. 16. Axial view showing appropriate placement of biotenodesis screw. (*From* Decarbo WT, Hyer CF. Interference screw fixation for flexor hallucis longus tendon transfer for chronic Achilles tendonopathy. J Foot Ankle Surg 2008;47(1):71; with permission.)

Tendinosis

Tendinosis is a chronic degenerative process with an inadequate reparative response. It is accompanied by collagen degeneration, fiber disorientation, scattered vascular ingrowth, and paucity of inflammation. Occasional necrosis or calcification can be found within the tendon. Pathologic studies have demonstrated morphologic changes with a decreased number of organelles within tenocytes, a diminished level of muco-polysaccharides and glycoproteins, and a smaller diameter and density of collagen fibers. These changes lead to increased stiffness and loss of viscoelasticity predisposing the elderly population to injury secondary to repetitive microtrauma.

In contrast to paratenonitis, physical examination findings consistent with tendinopathy demonstrate a mobile nodule that accompanies excursion of the Achilles tendon.

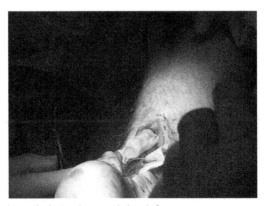

Fig. 17. The GraftJacket tabularized around the defect.

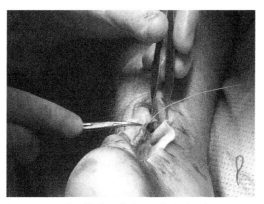

Fig. 18. The GraftJacket sewn to itself after being tabularized.

The nodule may or may not be tender to touch. The pathologic process lacks an inflammatory component and should not be associated with an increase of skin warmth or erytheme.

Maffulli and colleagues[52–55] studied biopsy specimens of patients with spontaneous subcutaneous Achilles rupture (27 men, 11 women; mean age 45.3 ± 13.8 years) and compared them to specimens of persons with no known tendon ailments (43 men, 3 women; mean age 64.2 ± 9.7 years). Using light microscopy, they noted a significantly greater amount of degeneration in the ruptured tendons with increased vascularity, decreased collagen stainability, hyalinization, and glycosaminoglycan. It was concluded that nonruptured Achilles tendons, even at an advanced age, and ruptured Achilles tendons are clearly part of two distinct populations.

Kannus[14] described lipoid and mucoid degeneration. Mucoid degeneration is represented by mucinous patches and vacuoles appearing brown or gray upon gross examination. Lipoid degeneration entails increased lipid deposition within the tendon.

Knobloch and colleagues[56] used power Doppler to evaluate the microcirculation of chronic Achilles tendinopathy. They demonstrated that significantly elevated microcirculatory blood flow occurs at the point of pain in insertional and midportion tendinopathy.

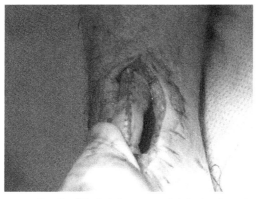

Fig. 19. Final repair once the GraftJacket is appropriately tensioned and sewn into the defect.

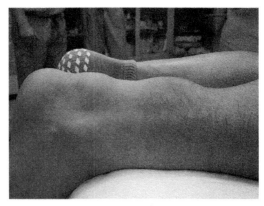

Fig. 20. Inflammatory reaction to equine xenograft (lateral view). (*Courtesy of* CF Hyer, DPM, Columbus, OH.)

Alfredson and colleagues[57,58] noted that glutamate, a well-known neurotransmitter and potent modulator of pain in the central nervous system, is found at high levels in the painful tendon. It is hypothesized that glutamate up-regulation occurs in conjunction with the neovascularization of chronic tendinopathy.

NONOPERATIVE TREATMENT FOR TENDINOSIS

One should avoid injecting the tendon because such an injection can cause iatrogenic rupture. Orthotics, boot walkers, and heel lifts may reduce symptoms by restoring mechanics of the foot and ankle, allowing rest and reducing tension on the Achilles. Occasionally, cast immobilization may be necessary. If symptoms resolve following a period of casting or immobilization in a boot, the patient can be slowly transitioned into a less conforming brace which can be worn in a shoe. Athletes returning to sport may benefit from a cross-training, starting with aquatics-based exercise.

Extracorporeal shock-wave therapy, similar to lithotripsy therapy for kidney stones, has proven to be an effective method of treatment for Achilles tendinopathy. It works via pressure change propagated through a liquid medium. It is theorized that

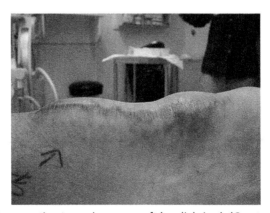

Fig. 21. Inflammatory reaction to equine xenograft (medial view). (*Courtesy of* CF Hyer, DPM, Columbus, OH.)

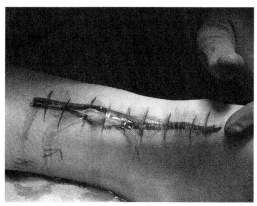

Fig. 22. Rush of inflammatory fluid following medial incision. (*Courtesy of* CF Hyer, DPM, Columbus, OH.)

increased blood flow alters the permeability of neuron cell membranes and induces inflammatory-mediated healing.[59,60]

Eccentric exercise training for Achilles tendinopathy has been studied since the 1980s. Proponents believe that it promotes collagen fiber cross-linking and facilitates remodeling. However, histologic evidence of this principle is lacking. Knobloch[56] published a prospective study to evaluate a 12-week eccentric training program and its effects on midportion and insertional tendinopathy. Knobloch concluded that eccentric training does not compromise tendon oxygen saturation. There was a significant decrease in capillary blood flow resulting in a reduction of pain.

Rompe and colleagues[61] performed a randomized control trial study evaluating the effect of eccentric loading versus the combination of eccentric loading and low-energy shock-wave treatment for midportion Achilles tendinopathy. They followed a series of 68 patients with chronic recalcitrant noninsertional Achilles tendinopathy (symptoms for a minimum of 6 months). The Victorian Institute of Sport Assessment—Achilles pain score validated for Achilles tendon problems was the outcome measurement tool. The investigators concluded that, at 4-month follow-up, the combined approach had a success rate of 82%, providing significantly better results than eccentric calf muscle training alone. At 1-year follow-up, there was no statistical difference between the two interventions.

SURGICAL TREATMENT

As a general rule, nonoperative measures should be exhausted before heading to surgery. Most investigators agree on at least 3 to 6 months of conservative treatment. Patients with isolated paratenonitis are at a low risk for tendon rupture. Those with tendinosis or a combination of tendinosis and paratenonitis are at a higher risk of rupture.

In cases where paratenonitis occurs in conjunction with tendonitis, the paratenon must be excised in addition to the area of tendinopathy. Whenever possible, a longitudinal incision is made within the tendon to shell out the diseased portion and then a longitudinal repair with tubularization is performed. When over one third of the tendon width is involved, some form of augmentation is indicated. Advanced imaging with ultrasound or MRI can help determine the extent of disease and aid in surgical planning. In severe cases that cannot be repaired, tendon transfers remain a viable alternative (**Fig. 23**).

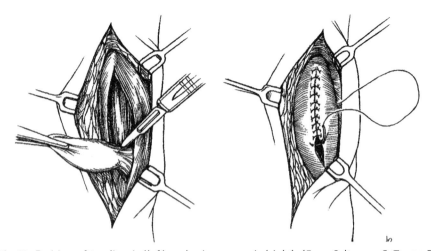

Fig. 23. Excision of tendinosis (*left*) and primary repair (*right*). (*From* Saltzman C, Tearse D. Achilles tendon injuries. J Am Acad Orthop Surg 1998;6(5):322; with permission. Copyright © 1998 American Academy of Orthopedic Surgeons.)

INSERTIONAL TENDINOPATHY

Insertional Achilles tendinopathy is associated with intrinsic tendon degeneration at the bone-tendon interphase. Baxter[62] reported that it is the most common form of tendinopathy in runners, with an incidence of 6.5% to 18%. Insertional Achilles tendinopathy is often diagnosed in older, less athletic, overweight individuals, and in older athletes. History reveals a slow dull aching pain in the posterior heel region that is exacerbated with activity. Athletes typically complain of increased pain affecting their ability to jump and run. Examination reveals tenderness at the tendon insertion with thickening or nodularity, and limited dorsiflexion of the ankle secondary to pain. It is not uncommon for a patient with insertional tendinopathy to have concomitant retrocalcaneal bursitis and a Haglund deformity.

Patients with retrocalcaneal bursitis are given a positive provocative examination by pressing from medial to lateral just anterior to the Achilles insertion. Those with a Haglund deformity have a posterolateral prominence of the calcaneus that causes direct tenderness and discomfort with footwear. When establishing the diagnosis of insertional tendinopathy, other causes of posterior heel pain, such as os trigonum, or posterior impingement should be ruled out.

Classically, overuse and poor training habits are considered to be the etiology of Achilles insertional tendinopathy. Myerson and McGarvey[63] have noted that a tight gastrocsoleus complex, hyperpronation, cavus foot, and obesity can predispose to degeneration, attrition, mechanical abrasion, and chemical irritation that could lead to a chronic inflammatory response to the heel.

Mafulli and colleagues[1] described the pathologic changes of insertional tendinopathy consisting of edema, mucoid degeneration, disruption of collagen bundles, necrosis, small hemorrhages, and calcification.

Radiographs can reveal intratendinous calcification, tractions spurs, or Haglund deformity. MRI can be used to assess the amount of degeneration or inflammatory change of the Achilles tendon, and rule out concomitant pathology, such as retrocalcaneal bursitis or posterior impingement.

MRI STRATIFICATION FOR INSERTIONAL TENDINOPATHY

Nicholson, Berlet, and Lee[64–67] developed an MRI-based stratification system for patients with insertional tendinopathy. A retrospective analysis of 157 patients (47 operative cases) was performed to collect information on patient demographics, duration of symptom, and type of therapeutic intervention. For the operative group, both preoperative and postoperative hindfoot AOFAS were obtained, as well as preoperative MRI. Stir sequence MRI images of the Achilles tendon within 2 cm of its insertion were analyzed. Investigators concluded that patients with tenderness at the Achilles tendon insertion who demonstrate greater than 8 mm of insertional tendon thickening and intramural degeneration involving more than 50% width were likely to fail nonoperative intervention.

NONOPERATIVE TREATMENT FOR INSERTIONAL TENDINOPATHY

McGarvey and colleagues[3] reported that nonoperative management of insertional calcific Achilles tendinosis has a 70% to 90% success rate. Treatment consists of rest, ice, anti-inflammatory medications, activity, and shoe-wear modifications. Shoe-wear modification includes heel lifts, open-back shoes, or a Cam Walker to avoid pressure on the posterior heel. Physical therapy modalities, such as cold therapy, ultrasound, iontophoresis, and eccentric calf stretching, may provide some benefit, depending upon the severity and duration of disease.

SURGICAL TREATMENT FOR INSERTIONAL TENDINOPATHY

The surgical goals for insertional Achilles tendinopathy include the removal of degenerative tendon and associated calcification, excision of the inflamed retrocalcaneal bursa, and resection of the prominent posterior calcaneal prominence.[68–70] As a general rule, time to recovery is directly related to the duration of symptoms and concomitant pathology.

Kolodziej and colleagues[71] performed a cadaveric study to determine how much of the Achilles tendon complex can be debrided before instability occurs. They dissected 24 fresh-frozen human calcanei and clamped them to a jig with a sophisticated hydraulic material testing machine. Investigators were able to release 25% of the insertion at a time while applying cyclic load to failure. By studying the specimens, investigators were able to determine that the average height of insertion measured 20 mm, average width at the proximal aspect of insertion was 24 mm, and distally the average width was 31 mm. They concluded that superior-to-inferior resection offered the greatest margin of safety when performing a partial resection of the Achilles insertion. As much as 50% of the tendon can be resected before the incompetence develops (**Fig. 24**).

SURGICAL TECHNIQUES

Various approaches to insertional Achilles tendinosis have been described, including a medial J-shaped incision, lateral incision, combination of medial and lateral incisions, and a posterior midline incision. Using just a medial or lateral approach may limit exposure, leading to inadequate debridement or to wound complications secondary to extensive pressure on the skin with retractors.

Midline Incision for Insertional Tendinopathy

Calder and Saxby[72] performed a chart review of 52 heels treated for insertional Achilles tendinosis with a midline posterior longitudinal incision and excision of the

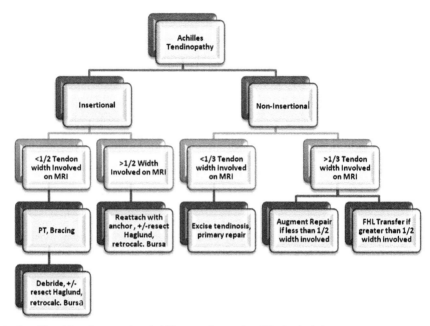

Fig. 24. Algorithm for treating Achilles tendinopathy. PT, physical therapy.

retrocalcaneal bursa, superior angle of the calcaneus, and diseased tendon. If greater than 50% of the cross-sectional area of the tendon was excised, then the tendon was augmented with suture anchors. Those with less than 50% involvement had a soft dressing applied and partial weight-bearing with crutches was initiated immediately after surgery. Ten to 14 days after surgery, patients were advanced to weight-bearing as tolerated. Those patients who had tendons that were more than 50% excised, and who had those tendons anchored, were initially placed in posterior splints. They were casted at their follow-up visit 10 to 14 days after surgery, and active physiotherapy was commenced at 6 weeks.

Investigators concluded that it is not necessary to immobilize all patients in a cast following surgery for those with less than 50% of the tendon excised. They attributed a small number of failures to inflammatory disorders, immunosuppressive medication, and weakness stemming from previous bilateral surgery. The investigators noted that failures were uncommon with the midline technique. They also related that a central tendon splitting approach might be safer because it avoids risk to neurovascular structures.

Johnson and colleagues[73] performed a retrospective study to evaluate the outcome of a central tendon splitting approach as described by McGarvey[3] for persistent insertional calcific Achilles tendinosis. The average duration of symptoms before surgical intervention was 3 years. Follow-up averaged 34 months (11–64 months). In general, approximately 50% to 70% of the Achilles insertion was estimated to have been released. Suture anchors were routinely used to augment the tendon insertion after debridement. Outcomes measured included the hindfoot AOFAS, shoe-wear comfort, and return to work. They found a significant improvement of total ankle-hindfoot scale scores increased from 53 points preoperatively to 89 points postoperatively (maximum 100). Pain significantly improved from a mean score of 7 points preoperatively to a mean score of 33 points (maximum 40). Function significantly improved from a mean score of 36 points preoperatively to 46 postoperatively (maximum 50). Significant improvement was observed in each component of the functional assessment. Comparison of patients older or younger than 50 years of age demonstrated a nonsignificant overall difference in outcome. The study concluded that a central tendon splitting approach yielded good relief of pain with improved function, shoe wear, and ability to work.

Medial Incision with Detachment for Insertional Tendinopathy

Wagner and colleagues[74] did a retrospective study of 75 patients over 5 years. Two groups were identified: a nondetached group and a detached group. In the detached group extensive debridement, reattachment with suture anchors, and a proximal V-Y lengthening was performed. The surgical procedure entailed a medial J-shaped incision with the decision to detach made intraoperatively. Postoperative management included a cast for up to 8 weeks and then a removable boot with a 0.626-in heel lift for another 4 weeks in those with complete detachment. Debridement-only patients were immobilized in a walking boot with heel lift for up to 4 weeks, followed by heel lift alone. Physical therapy was initiated for motion and gastrocsoleus strengthening at 4 weeks in the nondetached group and 12 weeks in the detached group. Average follow-up was 47 months for the nondetached group and 33 months for the detached group. Outcomes measured included pain, activity limitation, gait change, walking distance, return to sport or work, and level of satisfaction. Investigators found no statistically significant differences in the items evaluated (pain, limitations requiring an assistive device, gait, walking distance, ability to walk on uneven ground, ability to jump, ability to do deep knee bends, flexibility, use of any form of support or insert, ability to wear a closed-back shoe, return to sports or work). In the nondetached group, the satisfaction rate was 92% with 8% dissatisfied. In the detached group, 74% were completely satisfied, 18% with reservation, and 8% dissatisfied. Complications included minor wound dehiscence, wound infection, and sural neuritis.

Lateral Incision for Insertional Tendinopathy with Haglund Deformity

A lateral incision is used for a prominent posterolateral Haglund deformity. As always, caution is exercised when handling the soft tissue envelope. Dissection is carried down sharply to the calcaneal tuberosity with care to avoid the sural nerve. Once the Achilles tendon is identified, a distal longitudinal cuff of tendon is reflected laterally to enhance closure. The tendon is then gently reflected off the tuberosity from superior to inferior to expose the spur for resection. Once angled resection is performed, the edges should be smoothed with a rasp. Fluoroscopy can be used to ensure adequate decompression and to avoid leaving remnants of bone behind. Following decompression, closure is performed with a no-touch technique (**Figs. 25** and **26**).

Watson, Anderson, and Davis[75] reported the evaluation of 16 feet with retrocalcaneal bursitis and 20 feet with calcific Achilles insertional tendinosis that underwent retrocalcaneal decompression after failed nonoperative treatment. All of the surgeries were performed through a lateral approach with a retrocalcaneal bursectomy and, when indicated, excision of a calcific spur. Outcomes measured included ankle-hindfoot subscale AOFAS, satisfaction, time until maximum symptomatic improvement, and change demonstrated in radiographs. They noted that patients with calcific Achilles insertional tendinosis were older, required nearly twice the time to reach maximal symptomatic improvement (10.6 months compared with 5.9 months in retrocalcaneal bursitis group [not statistically significant]), had lower satisfaction rates (53.1 compared with 58 in retrocalcaneal bursitis group [not statistically significant]), had a lower pain score (34.2 compared with 38.6 in retrocalcaneal bursitis group

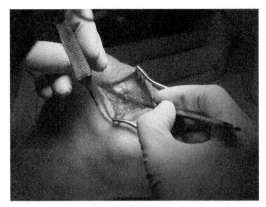

Fig. 25. Lateral approach to excising a Haglund deformity (identifying deformity.)

[statistically significant]), and had more shoe-wear restrictions. Radiographic recurrence did not correlate with outcome or symptomatic recurrence.

ARTHROSCOPIC DEBRIDEMENT OF INSERTIONAL ACHILLES TENDINOPATHY

Both Maquirriain[76] and Berlet[77] described an endoscopic technique for debridement of insertional Achilles tendinopathy. This technique allows for direct visualization and debridement of calcific enthesmophytes, retrocalcaneal bursa, Haglund deformity, and even reattachment of the Achilles to the tuberosity.

The procedure is performed in the prone position starting with medial portal placement adjacent to the Achilles at the level of the superior aspect of the calcaneus. A skin nick is carefully made followed by blunt dissection headed centrally to the retrocalcaneal space. A blunt dissector or freer is introduced through this portal and is used to carefully release the superior insertion, thus providing additional working area. Under direct visualization, a lateral portal is made adjacent to the Achilles. A 3.5-mm full-radius resector can then be used from either portal to provide further debridement and take down a Haglund deformity. Following the endoscopic procedure, the portals are closed and the patient is then placed in an equinus position and splinted. A boot walker with 1-in heel-lift is then initiated after 2 weeks.

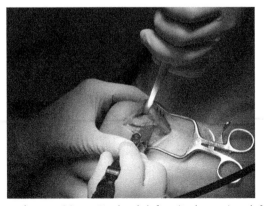

Fig. 26. Lateral approach to excising a Haglund deformity (removing deformity).

Limitations to the endoscopic technique include the presence of large intratendinous calcifications or large spurs that are difficult to remove through the scope. Also, extensive debridement and detachment may require more than one point of fixation into the calcaneal tuberosity.

SPORTS APPROACH FOR INSERTIONAL ACHILLES

For the young, competitive athlete with small insertional spurs, a tendon splitting approach may be most appropriate to allow minimal disruption of the Achilles with direct access to the spur and Achilles degeneration. A Haglund can be removed through this approach and the tendon interval repaired without having to use suture anchors. For the athlete with only a Haglund deformity and no spur or significant tendon involvement, an endoscopic approach can be particularly effective with little disruption of the Achilles insertion. An open small-incision approach directly over the Haglund (almost always lateral) can also be effective. For the older, active individual with large Haglund deformity, severe diffuse insertional Achilles tendon changes, and large extensive spurs, an open procedure with detachment of most of the Achilles insertion is necessary and can still allow a return to recreational sports. Typical return to sports is 3 months for the younger athlete with endoscopic or midline approach and 4 to 6 months for the older athlete with near complete reattachment.

SUMMARY

Achilles tendon disorders are common amongst the weekend warrior and active elderly patient population. The exact etiology remains unknown but it is most likely multifactorial. It is hypothesized that there is an association with overuse from repetitive loading. Histopathology has identified changes that occur with the aging tendon that may explain attritional ruptures without a definite trauma.

Thorough history and physical examination are key to developing the correct diagnosis. Advanced imaging is done to confirm the diagnosis, and may assist with surgical planning.

Aside from an acute full-thickness Achilles tendon rupture, most diagnoses can be initially treated nonoperatively. As a general rule, nonoperative measures should be exhausted before heading to surgery. One of the most common factors influencing prognosis and recovery with conservative treatment is duration of symptoms.

The common goal of both surgical and nonoperative management is to restore Achilles tendon function, reestablish a normal gait pattern, and relieve pain. Due to the risk of postoperative wound complications, those with significant medical comorbidities may be definitively treated with medications and bracing. Refinement in surgical technique has resulted in fewer postoperative complications with decreased rerupture rates and improved functional outcomes.

REFERENCES

1. Sayana MK, Maffulli N. Insertional Achilles tendinopathy. Foot Ankle Clin 2005;10: 309–20.
2. Saltzman C, Tearse D. Achilles tendon injuries. J Am Acad Orthop Surg 1998; 6(5):316–25.
3. McGarvey WC, Palumbo RC, Baxter DE, et al. Insertional Achilles tendinosis: surgical treatment through a central tendon splitting approach. Foot Ankle Int 2002;23:19–25.

4. Morelli V, James E. Achilles tendonopathy and tendon rupture: conservative versus surgical management. Prim Care 2004;31:1039–54.
5. Jozsal L, Kvist M, Balint BJ, et al. The role of recreational sport activity in Achilles tendon rupture. A clinical, pathoanatomical, and sociological study of 292 cases. Am J Sports Med 1989;17(3):338–43.
6. Bhandari M, Guyatt GH, Siddiqui F, et al. Treatment of acute Achilles tendon ruptures: a systematic overview and meta-analysis. Clin Orthop Relat Res 2002;400:190–200.
7. Cetti R, Christensen SE, Ijsted R, et al. Operative versus non-operative treatment of Achilles tendon rupture. A prospective randomized study and review of the literature. Am J Sports Med 1993;21:791–9.
8. Carden DG, Noble J, Chalmers J, et al. Rupture of the calcaneal tendon: the early and late management. J Bone Joint Surg Br 1987;69:416–9.
9. Inglis AE, Sculco TP. Surgical repair of ruptures of the tendo Achilles. Clin Orthop 1981;156:160–9.
10. Hansen, ST. Trauma to the heel cord. Trauma to the foot and ankle. Chapter 84, 2355–60.
11. Haries, M. Oxford textbook of sports medicine. 2nd edition. New York: Oxford University Press; chapter 4.4.3.
12. Clain MR, Baxter DE. Achilles tendinitis. Foot Ankle 1992;13(8):482–7.
13. Archambauh JM, Wiley JP, Bray RC. Exercise loading of tendons and the development of overuse injuries. A review of the current literature. Sports Med 1995;20:77–89.
14. Kannus L. Histopathological findings in spontaneous tendon ruptures. Scand J Med Sci Sports 1997;7(2):113–8.
15. Silver RL, De la Garza J, Rang M. The myth of muscle balance: a study of relative strengths and excursions of normal muscles about the foot and ankle. J Bone Joint Surg Br 1985;67:432–7.
16. Sorosky B, Press J, Plastaras C, et al. The practical management of Achilles tendinopathy. Clin J Sport Med 2004;14(1):40–4.
17. Strauss EJ, Ishak C, Jazrawi L, et al. Operative treatment of acute Achilles tendon ruptures: an institutional review of clinical outcomes. Injury 2007;38:832–8.
18. Hufner TM, Brandes DB, Thermann H, et al. Long-term results after functional non-operative treatment of Achilles tendon rupture. Foot Ankle Int 2006;27(3):168–71.
19. Khan, et al. Treatment of acute Achilles tendon ruptures. J Bone Joint Surg Am 2005;87:2202–10.
20. Mandelbaum BR, Myerson MS. Achilles tendon rupture. A new method of repair. Am J Sports Med 1995;23:392–5.
21. Krackow KA, Thomas SC, Jones LC. A new stitch for ligament-tendon fixation. Brief note. J Bone Joint Surg Am 1986;68:764–6.
22. Watson TW, Jurist KA, Yang KH, et al. The strength of Achilles tendon repair: an in vitro study of the biomechanical behavior in human cadaver tendon. Foot Ankle Int 1995;16(4):191–5.
23. Wong MWN, Ng VWS. Modified flexor hallucis longus transfer for Achilles insertional rupture in elderly patients. Clin Orthop Relat Res 2005;431:201–6.
24. Suchak A, Geoff P, Lauren A, et al. The influence of early weight-bearing compared with non-weight-bearing after surgical repair of the Achilles tendon. J Bone Joint Surg Am 2008;90:1876–83.
25. Teuffer AP. Traumatic rupture of the Achilles tendon. Reconstruction by transplant and graft using the lateral peroneus brevis. Orthop Clin North Am 1974;5(1):89–93.

26. Turco VJ, Spinella AJ. Achilles tendon ruptures—peroneus brevis transfer. Foot Ankle 1987;7(4):253–9.
27. Ma GWC, Griffith TG. Percutaneous repair of acute closed ruptured Achilles tendon: a new technique. Clin Orthop Relat Res 1977;128:47–55.
28. Maffulli N. Current concepts review. Rupture of the Achilles tendon. J Bone Joint Surg Am 1999;81(7):1019–35.
29. Hockenbury RT, Johns JC. A biomechanical in vitro comparison of open versus percutaneous repair of tendon Achilles. Foot Ankle 1990;11:67–72.
30. Hope M, Saxby TS. Tendon healing. Foot Ankle Clin 2007;12:553–67.
31. Lim J, Dalal R, Waseem M. Percutaneous vs. open repair of the ruptured Achilles tendon—a prospective randomized controlled study. Foot Ankle Int 2001;22(7): 559–65.
32. Lynn TA. Repair of the torn Achilles tendon, using the plantaris tendon as a reinforcing membrane. J Bone Joint Surg Am 1966;48(2):268–72.
33. Assal M, Jung M, Stern R, et al. Limited open repair of Achilles tendon ruptures: a technique with a new instrument and findings of a prospective multicenter study. J Bone Joint Surg Am 2002;84(2):161–70.
34. Barber FA, McGarry JE, Herbert MA, et al. A biomechanical study of Achilles tendon repair augmentation using GraftJacket matrix. Foot Ankle Int 2008; 29(3):329–33.
35. Clancy WG, Neidhart D, Brand RL. Achilles tendinitis in runners: a report of five cases. Am J Sports Med 1976;4(2):46–57.
36. Bosworth DM. Repair of defects in the tendo Achilles. J Bone Joint Surg Am 1956; 38(1):111–4.
37. Alfredson H. Conservative management of Achilles tendinopathy: new ideas. Foot Ankle Clin 2005;10:321–9.
38. Alfredson H, Cook J. A treatment algorithm for managing Achilles tendinopathy: new treatment options. Available at: www.bjsportmed.com. Accessed December 20, 2008.
39. Ronel DN, Newman MI, Gayle LB, et al. Recent advances in the reconstruction of complex Achilles tendon defects. 2003. Wiley InterScience Available at: www.interscience.wiley.com. Accessed December 20, 2008.
40. Christensen I. Rupture of the Achilles tendon. Analysis of 57 cases. Acta Chir Scand 1953;106(1):50–60.
41. Abraham E, Pankovich AM. Neglected rupture of the Achilles tendon treatment by V-Y tendinous flap. J Bone Joint Surg Am 1975;57(2):253–5.
42. Mann RA, Holmes GB, Seale KS, et al. Chronic rupture of the Achilles tendon: a new technique of repair. J Bone Joint Surg Am 1981;73(2):214–7.
43. Hahn F, Meyer P, Maiwald C, et al. Treatment of chronic Achilles tendinopathy and ruptures with flexor hallucis tendon transfer: clinical outcome and MRI findings. Foot Ankle Int 2008;29(8):794–802.
44. Hamish DH, Leslie MB, Edwards WHB. Neglected ruptures of the Achilles tendon. Foot Ankle Clin 2005;10:357–70.
45. Wapner KL, Pavlock GS, Hecht PJ, et al. Repair of chronic Achilles tendon rupture with flexor hallucis longus tendon transfer. Foot Ankle 1993;14(8): 443–9.
46. Pearsall AW, Bryant GK. A new technique for augmentation of repair of chronic Achilles tendon rupture. Foot Ankle Int 2006;27(2):146–7.
47. Decarbo WT, Hyer CF. Interference screw fixation for flexor hallucis longus tendon transfer for chronic Achilles tendonopathy. J Foot Ankle Surg 2008; 47(1):69–72.

48. DeOrio MJ, Easley ME. Surgical strategies: insertional Achilles tendinopathy. Foot Ankle Int 2008;29(5):542–50.
49. Feibel JB, Bernacki BL. A review of salvage procedures after failed Achilles tendon repair. Foot Ankle Clin 2003;8:105–14.
50. Cottom JM, Hyer CF, Berlet GC, et al. Flexor hallucis tendon transfer with an interference screw for chronic Achilles tendinosis: a report of 62 cases. Foot Ankle Specialists 2008;1(5):280–7.
51. Puddu G, Ippolito E, Postacchini F. A classification of Achilles tendon disease. Am J Sports Med 1976;4(4):145–50.
52. Maffulli N, Barress V, Ewen SW. Light microscopic histology of Achilles tendon ruptures. A comparison with unruptured tendons. Am J Sports Med 2000;28(6):857–63.
53. Maffulli N, Ewen SW, Waterston SW, et al. An in vitro model of human tendon healing. Am J Sports Med 2000;28(4):499–505.
54. Maffulli N, Testa V, Capasso G, et al. Calcific insertional Achilles tendinopathy, reattachment with bone anchors. Am J Sports Med 2004;32(1):174–82.
55. Maganaris CN, Narici MV, Maffulli N. Biomechanics of the Achilles tendon. Disabil Rehabil 2008;30(20–22):1542–7.
56. Knobloch K. Eccentric training in achilles tendinopathy: Is it harmful to tendon microcirculation? Br J Sports Med 2007. Available at: www.bjsportmed.com/cgi/content/full/41/6/e2. 1–5. Accessed December 20, 2008.
57. Alfredson H, Forsqrens, Thorsen K, et al. In vivo microdialysis and immunohistochemical analyses of tendon tissue demonstrated high amounts of free glutamate and glutamate receptors, but no signs of inflammation in jumper's knee. J Orthop Res 2001;19:881–6.
58. Angermann P, Hovgaard D. Chronic Achilles tendinopathy in athletic individuals: results of nonsurgical treatment. Foot Ankle Int 1999;20(5):304–6.
59. Furia JP. High energy extracorporeal shock wave therapy as a treatment for insertional Achilles tendinopathy. Am J Sports Med 2006;34(4):733–40.
60. Gallant GG, Massie C, Turco VJ. Assessment of eversion and plantar flexion strength after repair of Achilles tendon rupture using peroneus brevis tendon transfer. Am J Orthop 1995;24(3):257–61.
61. Rompe JD, Furia J, Maffulli N. Eccentric loading versus eccentric loading plus shock-wave treatment for midportion Achilles tendinopathy. A randomized controlled trial. Am J Sports Med 2009;37(3):463–70.
62. Baxter DE, Zingas C. The foot in running. J Am Acad Orthop Surg 1995;3:136–45.
63. Myerson MS, McGarvey W. Disorders of the Achilles tendon insertion and Achilles tendinitis. Instr Course Lect 1999;48:211–8.
64. Nicholson CW, Berlet GC, Lee TH. Prediction of the success of nonoperative treatment of insertional Achilles tendinosis based on MRI. Foot Ankle Int 2007;28(4):472–7.
65. Nigg BM. The role of impact forces and foot pronation; a new paradigm. Clin J Sport Med 2001;11(1):2–9.
66. Nilsson-Helander K, Swiird L, Silbernagel KG, Thomee R, et al. A new surgical method to treat chronic ruptures and reruptures of the Achilles tendon. Knee Surg Sports Traumatol Arthrosc 2008;16:614–20.
67. Pajala A, Kangas J, Ohtonen P, et al. Following treatment of total Achilles tendon rupture. J Bone Joint Surg Am 2002;84(11):2016–21.
68. Yodlowski ML, Scheller AD, Minos L. Surgical treatment of Achilles tendinitis by decompression of the retrocalcaneal bursa and the superior calcaneal tuberosity. Am J Sports Med 2002;30(3):318–21.

69. Young JS, Kumta SM, Maffulli N. Achilles tendon rupture and tendinopathy: management of complications. Foot Ankle Clin 2005;10:371–82.
70. Zanetti M, Metzdorf A, Kundert HP, et al. Achilles tendons: clinical relevance of neovascularization diagnosed with power Doppler US. Radiology 2003;227: 556–60.
71. Kolodziej P, Gisson RR, Nunley JA. Risk of avulsion of the Achilles tendon after partial excision for treatment of insertional tendonitis and Haglund's deformity: a biomechanical study. Foot Ankle Int 1999;20(7):433–7.
72. Calder JDF, Saxby TS. Surgical treatment of insertional Achilles tendinosis. Foot Ankle Int 2003;24(2):119–21.
73. Johnson KW, Zalavras C, Thordarson DB. Surgical management of insertional calcific Achilles tendinosis with a central tendon splitting aproach. Foot Ankle Int 2006;27(4):245–50.
74. Wagner E, Gould JS, Kneidel M, et al. Technique and results of Achilles tendon detachment and reconstruction for insertional Achilles tendinosis. Foot Ankle Int 2006;27(9):677–84.
75. Watson AD, Anderson RB, Davis HW. Comparison of results of retrocalcaneal decompression for retrocalcaneal bursitis and insertional Achilles tendinosis with calcific spur. Foot Ankle Int 2000;21(8):639–42.
76. Maquirriain J. Endoscopic Achilles tenodesis: a surgical alternative for chronic insertional tendinopathy. Knee Surg Sports Traumatol Arthrosc 2007;15:940–3.
77. Berlet G, Smith B, Giza E. Arthoroscopic retrocalcaneal burssectomy. In: Philbin T, editor. Surgical techniques in orthopaedics: Achilles tendon disorders. Special edition DVD. Rosemont (IL): American Academy of Orthopaedic Surgeons; 2008.

Management of Unstable Ankle Fractures and Syndesmosis Injuries in Athletes

J. Adam Jelinek, MD, David A. Porter, MD, PhD*

KEYWORDS

- Ankle • Unstable • Athletes
- Open reduction internal fixation
- Management • Ligament sports

The foot and ankle absorb tremendous stress during athletic competition. As a weight-bearing joint, the ankle can experience a multitude of different forces, reaching up to six times the athlete's body weight during vigorous activity.[1] Depending on the sport, a large amount of energy can be imparted across the ankle joint, leading to fracture and ligament disruption. These injuries can contribute to increased recovery time and more time loss before return to athletic activity. It has been estimated that between 15% and 25% of all athletic injuries involve the ankle.[2–4]

The treatment of ankle fractures and ligament injuries in the general population has been well documented. Treatments described in the literature range from a spectrum of conservative management with nonoperative immobilization to open reduction and internal fixation (ORIF) with hardware, depending on the injury type and soft tissue concerns. There are many components that determine the long-term success of treatment after ankle injury. The key factor is anatomic alignment of the ankle joint and complete healing, regardless of treatment method.[5–9] Ramsey and Hamilton[10] demonstrated that malunion of an ankle fracture leads to abnormal pressure distribution and eventual arthritis. The ultimate goal for outcome in treatment of an ankle fracture includes maintenance of a congruent joint, fracture union, functional motion, normal strength, and optimal recovery time. Operative stabilization of ankle fractures offers the potential for more rapid recovery than nonsurgical management.[7,11–17] Other factors involved in fracture management include the type of fracture,[6,7] joint surface alignment, patient age,[18,19] bone quality, and associated cartilage injury.[18,19]

Methodist Sports Medicine/The Orthopaedic Specialists Center, 201 Pennsylvania Parkway, Suite 200, Indianapolis, IN 46280, USA
* Corresponding author.
E-mail address: dporter@methodistsports.com (D.A. Porter).

Foot Ankle Clin N Am 14 (2009) 277–298
doi:10.1016/j.fcl.2009.03.003

Translation of ankle fracture management from the general population to the athlete may be problematic for a variety of reasons. First, the athlete typically has a robust skeletal system and a healthy soft tissue envelope that can provide a framework for rigid anatomic repair without soft tissue compromise. Next, the athlete imposes more demand on his or her ankle during competition than most nonathletes. Full strength and motion are required of the athlete before allowing safe return to sport, and the end point for outcome is typically return to unrestricted high-demand sport activity. These demands require careful detailed attention to functional strength and full range of motion (ROM). Finally, the athlete has additional concern regarding the time course to full return to sport, amount of immobilization required, and ability to rehabilitate while in the recovery stage. Despite the studies published describing ankle fractures and associated ligament injuries in the general population, the literature is sparse regarding the ideal treatment of ankle fractures and associated ligament injuries in the athlete.

Rigid anatomic surgical fixation of the athlete's unstable ankle injury reduces the concern for displacement while allowing early motion and weight bearing. Rigid fixation, in fact, allows range of movement (ROM) and weight bearing within 1 to 2 weeks of fixation, thus affording the athlete the opportunity to begin the rehabilitative process within days after injury and treatment.[11,20] The athlete is provided the opportunity to recover efficiently and rehabilitate simultaneously. Athletes treated with delayed weight bearing and prolonged immobilization require a longer time to achieve full ROM and strength, and thus delay return to sport.

The authors believe that athletes with the most unstable ankle injuries can return to their preinjury level of participation in 1 to 4 months with minimal functional morbidity and pain if they undergo rigid anatomic fixation followed by early motion and appropriate early weight bearing.[11]

ANATOMY

The ankle is a modified hinge joint. Motion occurs through a complex interaction of joint surfaces from the tibia, fibula, and talus, in addition to ligamentous restraint and dynamic muscle control. Rather than simple dorsiflexion and plantar flexion in the sagittal plane, coupled rotations occur in the axial and coronal planes.[21]

The deltoid ligament provides strong medial support to the ankle and is divided into superficial and deep portions. The superficial deltoid (also called the anterior deltoid) extends from the anterior colliculus and inserts onto the navicular, talus, and sustentaculum tali of the calcaneus.[22] The function of the superficial deltoid is primarily to resist external rotation of the talus and secondarily hindfoot eversion. The deep deltoid extends from the intercollicular notch of the medial malleolus and posterior colliculus to the medial talus (**Fig. 1**). Deep deltoid fibers are oriented transversely and form from a condensation of capsular fibers (see **Fig. 1**) that function primarily to prevent hindfoot eversion and secondarily to prevent external rotation of the talus. The deep deltoid is the primary soft tissue restraint to medial opening.[23] Repair of the deltoid for structural ligamentous stability must include the deep portion of the ligament. Even though this can be technically difficult, it is paramount to providing adequate stability. Isolated rupture of the anterior or superficial deltoid can occur and allows excess external rotation of the talus, but eversion is still restrained by the deep deltoid and the medial side can functionally still be stable.

The syndesmosis is made up of four ligaments and the interosseous membrane. It functions to hold the distal ends of the tibia and fibula together. The four ligaments include the anteroinferior tibiofibular ligament, the smaller posteroinferior tibiofibular ligament, the inferior transverse ligament, and the interosseous ligament. The

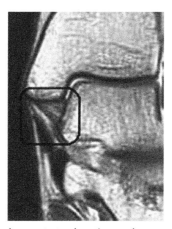

Fig. 1. Coronal view of ankle demonstrates location and anatomy of deep deltoid ligament (encircled deep deltoid, showing fibers from the tip of the medial malleolus to the medial talus).

interosseous ligament (also called the interosseus membrane) is the strongest portion of the syndesmosis and is the main ligamentous support between the tibia and fibula.[23] The syndesmosis and deltoid ligament help to stabilize talar position within the ankle joint by stabilizing the distal tibial-fibular joint complex. Anatomic fibular length and rotation are necessary for normal syndesmotic function and talar position within the ankle mortise.

Normal motion exists between the distal tibia and fibula. The fibula can move (although in small increments) medially, laterally, proximally, and distally, and it also has a rotational component in relation to the tibia. Fractures around the ankle and ligamentous disruptions can alter the normal mechanics and alignment of the ankle joint, leading to instability, altered contact pressures, pain, and functional instability. Thus, strict anatomic alignment and position are required for the athlete to return to full activity with full painless ROM.

HISTORY

A detailed history is required to determine the mechanism of these athletic injuries. Because many of these injuries or ankles can appear similar on initial presentation, an understanding of the mechanism of injury is crucial. A grade III lateral ankle sprain (which is treated with out surgery) can look similar to an unstable syndesmosis (treated with surgery). The mechanism of injury is the first guiding point toward differentiating. Location of injury, type of sport, position of the limb, direction of deforming forces, and magnitude and speed of injury are also important in the initial assessment. Elapsed time from initial injury allows the treating physician to correlate with the amount of swelling and aid in timing for potential operative management. Ability (or inability) to bear weight after the injury can be a clue to the significance of the injury. With unstable syndesmosis and bimalleolar ankle fracture injuries, the athlete is reluctant to bear weight, whereas an athlete with a grade III lateral sprain or an isolated lateral malleolus often can "walk" into the office or feel "stable" on the sidelines. Preinjury status of the extremity is also important in the initial evaluation. A lack of prior injury and totally normal function set the expectation for the athlete, although prior instability, spurring, or osteochondral lesions may need to be addressed concurrently with stabilization surgery. Concurrent, or prior, associated injuries can require the athlete to adjust his or her expectation of recovery and its timing. Although not as commonly helpful as in the general population, a general medical screen is still required, including questions regarding diabetes, vascular disease, neuropathy, alcohol use, and medication use. This screening process can uncover conditions that affect the timing of surgical intervention and the rehabilitation course, such as length of immobilization, concerns for soft tissue, risk for infection, and compliance.

PHYSICAL EXAMINATION

With any suspected ankle injury, a thorough examination of the extremity, including the skin integrity, neurovascular status, and associated soft tissue structures, should be performed. On physical examination, soft tissue edema, ecchymosis, and tenderness to direct palpation of the medial or lateral malleolus, the syndesmosis, and the deltoid guide the treating physician regarding the anatomic structures injured and the extent of injury. The entire fibula must be palpated to rule out proximal Maisonneuve type injury (proximal fibula fracture with syndesmosis and deltoid rupture). Pain and swelling over the soft tissue structures of the ankle complex, including the syndesmosis, lateral ligaments, and deltoid ligament, need careful, detailed, and discreet palpation. Even without obvious disruption, if the injury involved external rotation with abduction and significant ankle or lower leg swelling, a heightened suspicion for deltoid and syndesmosis injuries should remain. The deep deltoid ligament (partially intra-articular; see **Fig. 1**) and the posterior syndesmotic ligaments are structures deep within the ankle and can be difficult to palpate independently of other overlying and nearby structures. Each may be ruptured without isolated palpable tenderness. It can be difficult in the acute setting to be certain which of the structures are painful, even with careful and precise palpation. Therefore, follow-up evaluations can be warranted to determine the full extent of injury and differentiate between stable and unstable injuries. Repeat examinations and, occasionally, repeat radiographs together may finally be needed to understand the full and correct diagnosis. This is especially true with deltoid and syndesmosis injuries. To differentiate between an isolated anterior deltoid rupture and a complete deltoid rupture (anterior and deep) or between a high-grade but stable grade I syndesmosis and an occultly unstable grade II syndesmosis injury, these careful repeat evaluations may be required. The stakes are high in this differentiation, especially with the syndesmosis injury. A missed unstable syndesmosis injury that is undertreated can lead to a poor result and, potentially, career-ending disability.

Other important physical examination findings include provocative stress testing. The anterior drawer and talar tilt tests help in evaluation of lateral ligament stability. Pain with external rotation or with eversion is suggestive of syndesmosis or deltoid ligament injury and possible tear. The authors have not found the squeeze test to be reliable for evaluation of the syndesmosis.

Complete tears of the deltoid and syndesmosis and fractures present with significant swelling with medial or lateral ecchymosis, whereas stable syndesmosis, grade I ankle sprains, and nonfractures may have pain but do not have significant swelling or ecchymosis.

As with any documented ankle injury, regional structures, including the foot and, occasionally, the knee, must be evaluated. Particular attention to the foot should be given to rule out fractures of the anterior process of the calcaneus, the navicular, the lateral process of the talus, the base of the fifth metatarsal, the talar head, and ligamentous injuries of the midfoot (Lis franc).[1] Although it is uncommon to have significant ankle injuries with concomitant foot fractures or Lis franc disruption, it does occur. The authors treated a division I football player with a concomitant bimalleolar equivalent ankle fracture and a complete disruption of his Lis franc, which required operative fixation of both. Differentiating between severe foot injuries (Lis franc or lateral process fracture) and unstable ankle injures can be surprisingly challenging. The authors hope this article helps you in your evaluation.

RADIOGRAPHIC EVALUATION

Radiographs of the ankle are mandatory to evaluate bony and ligamentous injury. Information regarding mechanism of injury, severity of injury, best approach to the injury, and treatment can be ascertained with appropriate radiographs.[23] Anterior-posterior (AP), lateral, and mortise oblique radiographs are necessary to diagnose and classify the ankle injury. Foot radiographs can be taken if a concomitant injury is suspected lower than the ankle. The authors' radiographic series is taken with the patient standing (if at all possible) to allow for physiologic stress on the ligaments to help evaluate for occult deltoid and syndesmotic ligamentous injuries. This helps to differentiate between an isolated lateral malleolus fracture and a bimalleolar equivalent injury and between grade I and grade II syndesmosis injury. Manual stress radiographs (eversion and external rotation) are occasionally needed to evaluate occult deltoid or syndesmosis ruptures. Occult unstable syndesmosis injuries may require local anesthetic to obtain an adequate stress view. The authors use 1% lidocaine in the deltoid (3–5 mL) and distal syndesmosis (4–6 mL). For stressing the syndesmosis, external rotation with slight dorsiflexion oblique stress views is used to evaluate for occult instability with comparison made to the opposite side.

Evaluation of syndesmosis injuries by measuring diastasis of the tibia-fibula interval and tibia-fibula overlap on standard radiographs has not been as reliable in the authors' experience. The accuracy and reliability of measurements seem in question to the authors because of multiple variables, including rotation at the time the radiograph is taken, bony anomalies, and fibular notch size. There is still applicability in viewing the AP and oblique views of the ankle for the relation between the fibula and tibia; the authors do not rely on these findings as strongly to make their determination regarding stability, however. Medial clear space is used in their practice as the principal indicator of medial stability, and thus syndesmosis instability if the clinical picture is consistent (eg, external rotation injury, tenderness in syndesmosis, pain with external rotation test). With the ankle in neutral rotation, widening of the medial clear space greater than 1 to 2 mm more than the corresponding tibial-talar interval is highly suggestive of instability. Radiographic evaluation with full-length views of the tibia and fibula is needed to evaluate pronation or external rotation injuries resulting in a Maisonneuve type fracture (proximal fibula fracture with syndesmosis rupture).[24]

CLASSIFICATION

The two most common classification systems for skeletally mature ankle fractures include the Danis-Weber (A.O. Müller) and Lauge-Hansen classification systems. Isolated lateral malleolar fractures are classified according to the Danis-Weber classification system. A Danis-Weber type A fracture involves a fracture of the fibula lower than the level of the tibial plafond (**Fig. 2**). A Danis-Weber type B fracture involves an oblique or spiral fracture at or near the level of the ankle joint caused by an external rotation mechanism (**Fig. 3**). Type C injuries involve a fracture higher than the level of the ankle joint (**Fig. 4**). The more proximal the fibular fracture, the greater is the risk for syndesmosis disruption and associated instability. The Lauge-Hansen classification system describes four distinct injury patterns, based on cadaveric studies, which

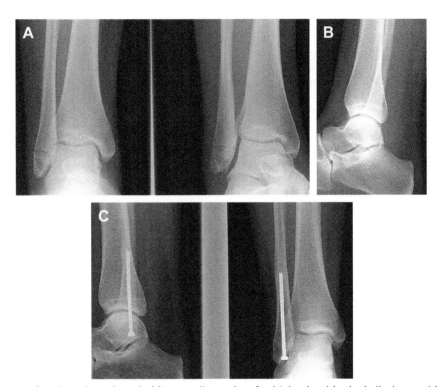

Fig. 2. (A, B) AP, lateral, and oblique radiographs of a high-school basketball player with inversion and adduction injury attributable to a Weber A displaced fracture of the fibula. At the time of surgery, the periosteum was interposed within the fracture site, preventing anatomic reduction. (C) Postoperative radiographs demonstrate a 4.5-mm cannulated retrograde screw with anatomic reduction of the fracture.

take into account the position of the foot at the time of injury and the direction of the deforming force. This system describes pure injury sequences, with each injury pattern subdivided into stages of increasing severity. The four patterns include supination-adduction, supination-external rotation, pronation-abduction, and pronation-external rotation. The authors have found the supination-adduction class to be particularly helpful because it guides their approach to operative fixation. They use transverse screws medially (previously without a plate but more recently with a low-profile small distal tibia plate) and a retrograde 4.5-mm or 5.5-mm cannulated screw in the fibula to fix the Weber type A avulsion fracture (see **Fig. 2**).

The most commonly used classification of pediatric ankle fractures is the Salter-Harris anatomic system. This classification system, popularized because of its relative simplicity and ability to provide injury prognosis, divides injury patterns into grade I through grade V. The authors have found this classification system useful. Salter-Harris grade I injury is classified by physeal injury without radiographic evidence of bony injury, whereas grade II injury is characterized by a fracture line that extends transversely through the physis and exits proximally through the metaphysic (**Fig. 5**). Salter-Harris grade III injury involves a fracture that transverses the physis and exits distally through the epiphysis (**Fig. 6**). Grade IV injury is characterized by a fracture line that traverses the epiphysis and physis and exits the metaphysis, whereas a crush to the physis delineates a Salter-Harris grade V injury. Syndesmosis injuries involve

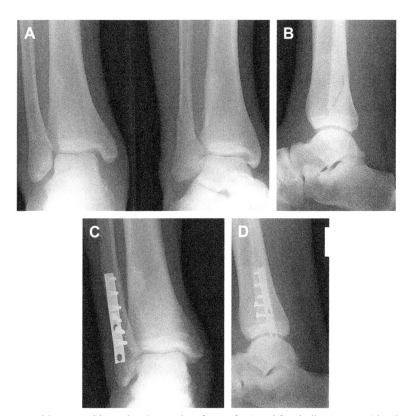

Fig. 3. AP, oblique, and lateral radiographs of a professional football receiver with a bimalleolar equivalent ankle fracture before (*A, B*) and AP and lateral radiographs after (*C, D*) operative fixation of fibula with an antiglide plate and primary repair of the deltoid ligament.

grades I through III. A grade I injury presents with normal alignment throughout the ankle, and the stability is maintained on stress views. A grade III injury shows widening of the medial clear space and, in most instances, widening of the tibia-fibula interval (**Fig. 7**). A grade II injury is more deceptive; it is stable on nonstressed views like a grade I injury but demonstrates widening and instability on stress views like a grade III injury.

GENERAL MANAGEMENT PRINCIPLES

Priorities for the ankle include assurance of adequate blood flow (pink color and palpable pulses), provisional reduction of marked deformity or dislocation if present (done in the emergency department or, occasionally, in the field if the physician is present), care of open wound or soft tissue injury, precise reduction of skeletal deformity through surgery if indicated, repair of associated injuries, rehabilitation, and, finally, care of any potential complications that develop. The authors believe that the best functional results are obtained with anatomic reduction of the fracture and joint surfaces, maintaining the reduction until healing, and joint mobilization as soon as possible without compromising reduction. Prolonged immobilization can result in

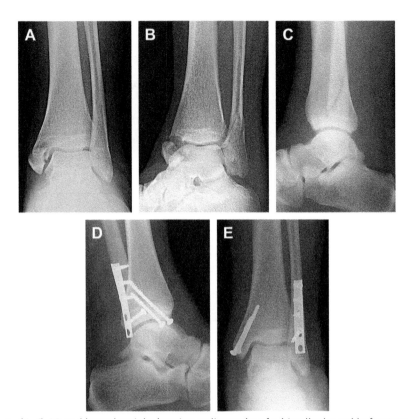

Fig. 4. (A–C) AP and lateral weight-bearing radiographs of a bimalleolar ankle fracture sustained in a 21-year-old collegiate diver. (D, E) Follow-up radiographs 1 week after stabilization.

poor results and undesired sequelae, including muscle atrophy, arthrofibrosis, cartilaginous degeneration, and bone atrophy.[23]

LATERAL MALLEOLAR FRACTURES

Surgical reduction and rigid internal fixation are recommended to athletes with isolated lateral malleolar fractures if displacement is greater than 2 to 4 mm or if there is significant external rotation or shortening. If the athlete prefers a more rapid yet safe return to sports and the fracture is displaced 2 to 4 mm, the authors offer operative fixation. Fixation is approached with general adherence to the Arbeitsgemeinschaft Fur Osteosynthesfragen (AO/ASIF) technique.

Porter and colleagues[11] recently reported on a series of 27 unstable ankle injuries treated by ORIF. The authors have treated Danis-Weber type A injuries with retrograde intramedullary 4.5-mm or 5.5-mm cannulated screw fixation after anatomic reduction (see **Fig. 2**). Danis-Weber type B injuries are treated with anatomic reduction, anterior-to-posterior lag screw fixation, and a posterolateral one-third semitubular antiglide plate (see **Fig. 3**). For Danis-Weber type C injuries, the authors stabilize the fibula with a lateral plate and, occasionally, a 2.7-mm or 3.5-mm lag screw (see **Fig. 4**). The thickness and length of the plate depend on the amount of comminution and length of

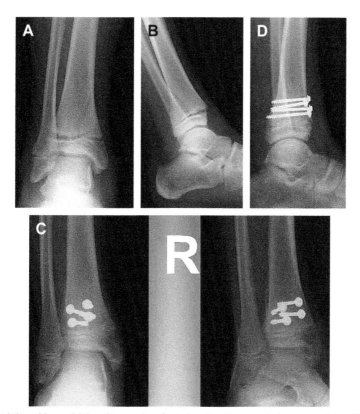

Fig. 5. AP (A) and lateral (B) radiographs of a Salter-Harris grade II fracture of the distal tibia in a 13-year-old competitive basketball player who landed awkwardly. AP, lateral, and oblique (C, D) postoperative radiographs of the patient after fixation with four 4.0-mm cannulated screws.

fracture. Often a one-third tubular plate is adequate; only rarely do the authors use a 3.5 low contour compression (LCDC) plate for the Weber C fractures. If the syndesmosis is unstable to external rotation stress after fixation, one to two 4.5-mm cannulated syndesmosis screws are inserted through the lateral fibular plate and across three cortices in the standard fashion (see **Fig. 4**).[11] The authors are currently looking at the possibility of using a standard tight rope in this setting to stabilize the syndesmosis but have no data on this approach. With fixation of the Weber type C fibula with a plate and screws, the degree of syndesmosis instability can be significant but still less than an unstable Maissoneuve type. Thus, a tight rope may provide adequate stabilization when there is a shorter segment of interosseus membrane disruption with these "low" fibular shaft fractures. A tight rope fixation for these short segment disruptions may allow stabilization without the need for hardware removal.

Athletes with isolated lateral malleolar fractures (Weber type A and B) demonstrate the most rapid return to sports. These athletes often rate their ankle as normal as early as 3 to 4 months after fixation, and four of the six athletes in the authors' study[11] still rated their ankle as 100% at 2 years after fixation. Stiffness and an occasional sense of giving away (likely attributable to the stiffness) are the most common complaints that the authors noted.[11] Because fracture healing has not been an issue, the authors focus

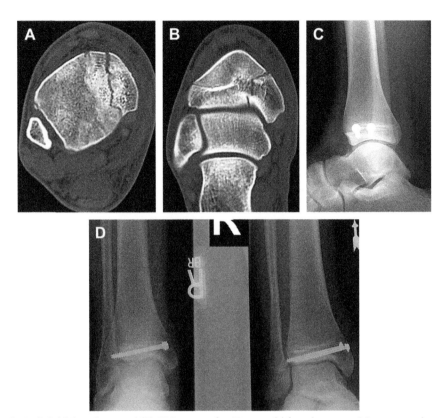

Fig. 6. Axial (*A*) and coronal (*B*) CT images of a 12-year-old female competitive soccer player who suffered a Salter-Harris grade III distal tibia fracture. (*C, D*) Soccer athlete underwent ORIF with two 4.0-mm cannulated screws of the Salter-Harris grade III fracture of the distal tibia. The hardware was subsequently removed.

especially on getting full ROM and full strength in their rehabilitation protocol. Early return to full activity (as early as 4 weeks) can occur with rigid antiglide fixation and accelerated rehabilitation with a stirrup brace support after coming out of the boot.

BIMALLEOLAR FRACTURES AND BIMALLEOLAR EQUIVALENT FRACTURES

The authors classify the true bimalleolar fracture (medial malleolus and lateral malleolus) and bimalleolar equivalent (lateral malleolus and deltoid rupture) together, because the prognosis, recovery, rehabilitation, and decision making are similar. Surgical stabilization is recommended for athletes with bimalleolar fractures or equivalent injuries because of the inherent instability with this injury pattern (see **Fig. 3; Fig. 8**). Standing and, occasionally, stress radiographs (preoperative or intraoperative) are used to establish the diagnosis and assess ligamentous integrity (deltoid). Confirmation of the deltoid ligament disruption as part of the bimalleolar equivalent injury is obtained at the time of surgery by stress fluoroscopy (wide medial clear space) and direct visualization (with repair).

Bimalleolar fractures require anatomic reduction and fixation of the fibula as described (antiglide for Weber type B, see **Fig. 3**; lateral side plate for Weber type C), in addition to reduction and fixation of the medial malleolus with lag screws (4.0-mm

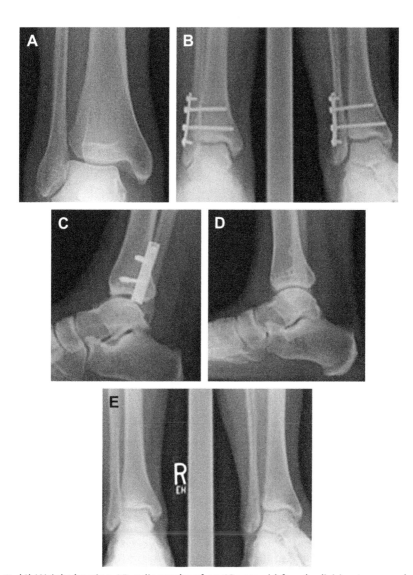

Fig. 7. (A) Weight-bearing AP radiographs of an 18-year-old female division I soccer player who sustained an unstable syndesmosis injury. (B, C) Weight-bearing radiographs taken 2 weeks after anatomic reduction and fixation of the syndesmosis injury. Hardware was removed at 3 months after initial fixation. (D, E) Weight-bearing radiographs at 7 months after initial surgery and after returning to competitive soccer.

partially threaded cancellous; see **Fig. 8**). Bimalleolar equivalent injuries were treated according to the protocol of Weber type B (see **Fig. 3**) or Weber type C fibula fractures, with additional direct repair of the deltoid ligament. The authors use two number 1 Vicryl horizontal mattress sutures in the deep deltoid and two 0 Vicryl sutures in the superficial (anterior) deltoid. In their classification system, for a Weber type C fibula in a bimalleolar pattern, the syndesmosis is stable and does not need fixation (see elsewhere in this article for syndesmosis rupture).

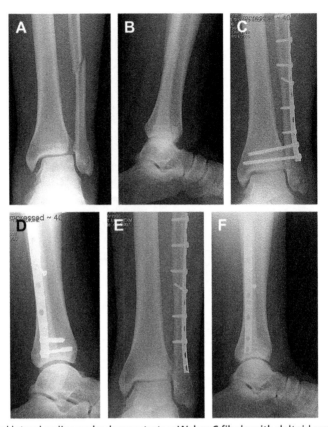

Fig. 8. AP and lateral radiographs demonstrate a Weber C fibula with deltoid rupture before surgery (*A, B*), after fixation with a one-third tubular plate and two 4.5-mm screws with repair of deltoid (*C, D*), and after removal of the two syndesmosis screws (*E, F*).

Recovery can be near normal for the athletes with bimalleolar fractures if there is normal cartilage (or only minor scuffing). The authors reported on 10 athletes classified and treated as having bimalleolar or bimalleolar equivalent fractures. Three athletes had true bimalleolar fractures, and 7 had bimalleolar equivalent injuries. Three of the 10 athletes rated their ankle at 100% on the Ankle Fracture Research Study questionnaire. Of the 7 athletes who did not rate their ankle at 100%, 5 cited occasional pain, 1 cited stiffness, 1 cited swelling, 1 cited decreased flexibility, and 1 cited fear of reinjury. Two athletes cited more than a single reason.[11] The overall rating from the 10 athletes was 97% with regard to pain and 92% with relation to function at 2 years after injury. Normal ankles rate out as 99% for pain and function.

UNSTABLE SYNDESMOSIS INJURIES

Unstable ankle syndesmosis injuries occur when the interosseus ligament is ruptured and disrupts the normal stabilization mechanism of the talus within the ankle mortise (see **Fig. 7**). Such injury requires fixation across the tibia and fibular joint to prevent excess motion and to allow the syndesmosis ligamentous complex to heal (see **Fig. 7**). Syndesmosis rupture is confirmed when there is widening of the medial clear space in association with widening of the tibia-fibula interval at the level of the ankle.

Unstable syndesmosis injuries, with or without a fibula fracture, are reduced with a large reduction clamp and a four-hole one-third tubular plate with two 4.5-mm can-nulated screws fixated across three cortices (see **Fig. 7**). Two 3.5-mm unicortical screws are placed in the proximal and distal holes of the lateral plate for positioning of the plate. If a fibula fracture was present, a one-third tubular plate long enough to stabilize the fracture was used in addition to standard syndesmosis fixation, as described previously (see **Fig. 4**). As a standard routine, syndesmosis screws were removed at approximately 3 months.[11]

Porter and colleagues[11] reported on the treatment of four athletes with distal tibial-fibular syndesmosis disruption. Three of the four athletes did not rate their ankle at 100% on the Ankle Fracture Research Study questionnaire. Two athletes cited reduced strength, and one athlete cited occasional pain as the reason for the reduced rating. The pain score for the whole group was 98%, and the function score was 97%, indicating near-normal function and minimal pain despite near-immediate weight bearing and minimal immobilization.

PHYSEAL INJURIES

With increased overall participation and a younger population of athletes taking part in sporting activities, it is not uncommon to see unstable ankle injuries in athletes with open physes. Pediatric ankle fractures account for 5% of pediatric fractures and 15% of physeal injuries. Peak incidence occurs between the age of 8 and 15 years, and the annual incidence of pediatric ankle fractures is approximately 0.1%.[25] Liga-mentous injuries are uncommon in this subgroup of athletes, because the ligaments are generally stronger than the open physes. Grossly displaced physeal injuries are initially treated with gentle closed reduction and immobilization in the emergency room or operating room setting to allow adequate pain control and more accurate reduction. Postreduction radiographs should be evaluated to assess adequacy of alignment of the physes and fracture. Traditionally, ORIF is used to decrease the risk for physeal arrest and to enhance articular congruity. Greater than 2 mm of residual displacement after closed reduction is a general indication for operative inter-vention.[25] The authors have noted in their young athletes that most of the injuries involve 3 to 8 mm of displacement at the physes and 2 to 5 mm at the articular surface. They typically recommend ORIF if the articular surface is displaced greater than 2 mm (see **Fig. 6**) or if the physes is displaced 3 to 4 mm or greater (see **Fig. 5**). Also, if there is any rotational or angular deformity, the authors recommend ORIF.

Salter-Harris type fractures that required surgery were reduced to an anatomic posi-tion and then fixated with 4.0-mm cannulated screws. Care was taken to avoid crossing the physis in each case (see **Figs. 5** and **6**).

In the study by Porter and colleagues,[11] four athletes were treated for Salter-Harris type fractures. Two athletes had an isolated Salter-Harris grade III fracture of the distal tibia, one athlete had a Salter-Harris grade III fracture of the distal tibia and fibula, and one athlete had a Salter-Harris grade IV fracture of the distal tibia and a Salter-Harris grade II fracture of the distal fibula. All four athletes rated their ankles at 100% on the Ankle Fracture Research Study questionnaire. Thus, with these young athletes, anatomic reduction of the physes and rigid fixation with screw(s) can lead to essen-tially normal results.

RESULTS

Porter and colleagues[11] reviewed 27 athletes with unstable ankle fractures fixed surgi-cally. The average age was 18 years, and the most common sports were football and baseball. Other sports leading to unstable ankle injuries included cheerleading, soft-ball, wrestling, basketball, gymnastics, motocross, rock climbing, rodeo, rugby, soccer, and volleyball. Average follow-up was 2.4 years. All follow-up radiographs demonstrated complete healing of the fracture, and the average percentage rating on the Ankle Fracture Research Study questionnaire was 96.4%. Twelve of the 27 athletes rated their ankle at 100%. Average motion was 82.7° of planar flexion, 15.8° of dorsiflexion, 17.6° of inversion, and 5.2° of eversion compared with 81°, 17.1°, 17.3°, and 4.6°, respectively, of the noninjured extremity. There were no signif-icant differences ($P>0.05$, ANOVA) in ankle ROM when compared with the contralat-eral uninjured side. For each ankle fracture type, postsurgical recovery time for use of rehabilitative devices and time required for resumption of activities were described **(Table 1)**.[11]

Of the 27 athletes treated with ORIF for unstable ankle injury, there were two cases of suspected infection. These two cases were treated with oral antibiotics for precau-tionary reasons. Both were in conjunction with syndesmosis screws, and all hardware was removed after 3 months. Cultures of tissue and hardware were negative for infec-tion. It does not seem that there was actually any bacterial infection but just a reaction to the syndesmosis screw. There were two cases of temporary numbness around the incision site and one case of temporary hypersensitivity to pain around the incision site. All three cases resolved without any permanent disability after 2 to 3 weeks.[11]

All athletes treated with ORIF for unstable ankle fractures were able to resume activ-ities of daily living and their previous level of competition, with one exception. One athlete, who sustained a bimalleolar ankle fracture, did not resume preinjury compet-itive activity because of fear of reinjury. No objective evidence supported the athlete's inability to return to full competition.[11] This is the only study the authors aware of that has reported on a series of ankle fractures in athletes. Donley and colleagues[26] re-ported on three professional football players with ORIF of ankle fractures. All three had pronation-external rotation injuries and rigid fixation, but these investigators did not report their patients' time to return to sports and had a less aggressive approach to rehabilitation.

Table 1
Time (in weeks) athletes required the use of rehabilitative devices and time when athletes were able to resume activities

Classification	N	Crutches	Boot	Brace	Daily Living	Practice	Competition
Lateral malleolus fracture	6	1.3 ± 0.5	3.0 ± 0.9	4.3 ± 3.8	1.2 ± 0.8	5.0 ± 0.9	6.8 ± 2.4
Medial malleolus fracture	2	2.0 ± 1.4	2.0 ± 1.4	7.0 ± 1.4	2.0 ± 0.0	12.0 ± 5.7	17.0 ± 9.9
Bimalleolar fracture and equivalent	10	3.7 ± 1.6	3.7 ± 2.0	4.2 ± 2.2	1.0 ± 0.5	10.9 ± 4.0	12.7 ± 4.0
Syndesmosis disruption injury	4	3.3 ± 1.0	2.3 ± 1.3	6.8 ± 6.1	0.8 ± 0.5	13.5 ± 2.5	15.8 ± 1.7
Salter-Harris type fracture	4	2.0 ± 0.8	3.5 ± 1.7	9.0 ± 1.2	1.0 ± 0.0	6.3 ± 1.3	8.5 ± 1.0
Pilon fracture	1	4.0	2.0	2.0	1.0	8.0	16.0

FUNCTIONAL REHABILITATION

The goal of rehabilitation is to obtain functional recovery and allow the athlete to return to sporting activity safely as quickly as possible. The intent of early ROM, weight bearing, and modified exercise is to incorporate rehabilitation of the ankle with the natural healing process of the ankle injury, and thus to accelerate the return to sports at a preinjury level.

Initial treatment of the postoperative ankle injury includes rest, ice, compression, and elevation. These modalities are useful to help decrease swelling and reduce pain. Pain is mediated through temperature by means of neurosynaptic pathways. It has been demonstrated that reducing the temperature in tissue leads to a decrease in sensory and motor nerve velocity, eventually blocking synaptic transmission of pain signals.[27] The decreased temperature of cryotherapy can also lead to arterial vasoconstriction, a decrease in local metabolism, and an elevated pain threshold. Elevation of the extremity can decrease hydrostatic pressure and results in edema reduction.[28] After surgery, the treating physician must monitor the use of cryotherapy in the setting of wet dressings, because this combination has the potential to decrease skin temperature to a dangerous level.

The goal of rigid anatomic internal fixation is to provide stability for early ROM and weight bearing. Early ROM provides the advantages of controlled ligament stress to stimulate strength, decreased risk for muscle atrophy and arthrofibrosis, and timely return to function. Ligaments often hypertrophy in response to early ROM to compensate for decreased tensile strength of the individual fibers. When implementing a rehabilitation program, the amount of tension and stress must not overcome the ultimate load to failure of the tissue and must not lead to fatigue of the ligament or plastic deformation.[28] The concept of early ROM has been borne out as being advantageous in the literature for flexor tendons of the hand[29–31] and anterior cruciate ligament reconstruction.[32] Salter and colleagues[33] demonstrated that early continuous passive motion on synovial joints allows and promotes cartilage nutrition and health. Passive ROM allows relaxation of the muscles while the joint is mobilized. Active ROM allows for muscle activation and incorporates re-education of the muscle. ROM must be tempered to work ROM in the direction opposite of the mechanism of injury until the ligament has healed. This protects the healing ligament during the recovery phase.

Early weight bearing, if possible given the specific injury pattern, is preferable and provides an advantage for the athlete. Early protected weight bearing has been shown to increase the stability of the lateral ankle ligaments. Other advantages of early weight bearing include decreased muscle atrophy, decreased joint stiffness, and decreased proprioception dysfunction. Trappe and colleagues[34] examined the effects of weight-lessness on muscles during a 17-day space flight. They found an 11% decrease in muscle power and a 21% decrease in muscle force at peak power velocity after just 17 days of weightlessness. Muscle fiber diameter also decreased, with a measured single fiber diameter decrease of 20%. They have also noted that non-weight bearing with crutches results in similar findings.

ROM must be achieved as the first step of the ankle rehabilitation process. Strengthening can be initiated once 95% to 100% of the preinjury ROM is achieved. An appropriate strengthening program includes isometric, isotonic (concentric and eccentric), and isokinetic exercises for the ankle after rigid fixation.

Proprioception, or the ability of the body to vary the forces of muscles in response to outside forces, is an important component in the successful rehabilitation of the athlete after ankle fracture. Proprioceptive input is provided through muscles, ligaments, tendons, and receptors within the joint. Injury alters the normal protective proprioceptive mechanisms in the extremity and must be rehabilitated to decrease the chance of continued or recurrent injury. Treatment regimens to improve proprioception include early weight bearing, double leg stance, and progressing to single leg stance. More advanced rehabilitation techniques for increasing proprioception include a biomechanical ankle proprioception system board or kinesthetic awareness trainer.

After injury, it is important to keep the athlete active from a cardiovascular, physical, and mental standpoint. Cardiovascular activities increase cellular metabolic levels and enhance blood flow to the healing extremity. The athlete should be engaged in the rehabilitation program rather than acting as a passive bystander. This can increase motivation and provides psychologic benefits during recovery.

Before return to sport after ankle fracture ORIF, a functional progression should be instituted. A functional progression is a series of sport-specific skills with a stepwise increase in the level of difficulty. The athlete must systematically progress and successfully complete each step without pain or apprehension before a safe return to competition. This provides physiologic and psychologic benefits to the athlete, maximizing confidence and decreasing apprehension for return to competition. The authors have found that if an athlete can complete the functional progression program after ankle fracture ORIF, he or she has been successful in returning to his or her sport.

Postoperative rehabilitation of unstable ankle injuries is divided into three phases. Each phase has specific goals, and advancement from one phase to the next depends on achieving these goals. Phase I provides an initial focus on the soft tissue inflammation and edema. This phase emphasizes pain control, decreasing inflammation, and restoration of normal joint ROM. Once these goals are accomplished, the patient is ready to progress to phase II. The focus of phase II is foot and ankle flexibility with functional strengthening. Cardiovascular conditioning, proprioceptive training, and light sport-specific functional training are initiated during this phase. Once these goals are completed and the athlete is ready for a gradual return to sporting activity, phase III is initiated. Phase III emphasizes return to normal function and preinjury sport-specific activity. Maintenance of flexibility and strength and teaching proper mechanics can help to ensure a safe return to sport. A functional progression is also implemented at this time before return to full functional participation. External supports, such as braces, straps, taping, and orthotics, may also be used to allow pain-free sport participation.[28] The authors require their athletes to wear a brace for their first season of participation after fixation for an ankle fracture and believe that it helps proprioception and confidence for the athlete.

Acute displaced fractures and ligament injuries treated by ORIF with the goal of rigid anatomic fixation can be advanced with a generalized functional rehabilitation program as described previously. A specific program can be initiated as follows.

Phase I

Immediately after surgery, the patient is placed in a walking boot (Aircast; DJO, Inc., Vista, California) with a Cryo/Cuff (Aircast; DJO Inc.) for cold and compression. Patients are instructed to rest, elevate the extremity, and use the Cryo/Cuff continuously during waking hours. To enhance circulation and decrease the risk for thrombosis, toe curls, leg lifts, and knee bends are instituted every 1 to 2 hours while awake. Patients are initially instructed to use axillary crutches and to maintain non–weight-bearing status.

At 1 week after surgery, dressings are changed to evaluate the wound and radiographs are taken. If stability is demonstrated on radiographs, a supervised home exercise program is initiated (or supervised by an athletic trainer if available), consisting of ROM exercises, toe curls, resistive band exercises, desensitization massage, and a light bike program in the boot. ROM and light tubing exercises should be performed several times per day at high repetitions (15–20 repetitions) and guided by pain. Stretching is also initiated if there is no contraindicating ligament injury, including towel stretch for the Achilles tendon and manual plantar flexion stretch (20 seconds, 5 repetitions). If there is a concomitant ligament injury, care is taken not to place undo stress on the repair during ROM exercises (the authors do not allow external rotation in first 6 weeks if there is deltoid repair). ROM is not limited for isolated fibula fractures or stable bimalleolar fractures. Dorsiflexion and eversion are avoided with a ruptured deltoid ligament until the ligament is healed, however.

If stability is radiographically confirmed at 1 week, partial weight bearing with axillary crutches is initiated in the boot with progression to full weight bearing at 2 weeks. Patients are progressed with two crutches initially, then with one crutch under the opposite arm, and, finally, with no assistive devices. The patient is weaned out of the boot into a stirrup brace and an athletic shoe over a 2-week period once he or she can walk without a limp in the boot, typically around 2 weeks after surgery for an isolated fibula fracture and 4 to 6 weeks after surgery for bimalleolar and syndesmosis injuries.[11,28] The athlete's bike program is progressed until he or she can ride a bike with the stirrup brace for 30 to 40 minutes per day without pain or discomfort (**Table 2**).[28] The athlete is instructed to wear the stirrup brace during all types of activity during the initial 2 to 6 weeks of recovery. After this initial period, the athlete is instructed to wear the brace only during athletic activity for 6 weeks with an isolated fibula fracture or Salter-Harris type fracture and for 3 months with a bimalleolar or syndesmosis injury.

Phase II

The time frame for the start of phase II depends on the individual patient's progress, but it generally begins approximately 1 month after surgery. The focus of phase II includes increased weight-bearing exercises, proprioception, and gait training with an athletic shoe. Resistive tubing exercises are progressed with continued high repetitions (15–20 repetitions) and can now include directions avoided previously because of concomitant ligament injury. New exercises initiated during this phase include standing calf stretching, balancing exercises, double to single leg calf raises, elliptic exercises, and stair-climbing exercises. Standing calf stretching should be performed

Table 2
Cardiovascular exercise program

	Exercise Equipment	Supportive Device	Minutes	Times per Week
Week 1	Stationary bike Stair climbing Elliptic	Boot Brace Shoe/insert	10	3
Week 2	Stationary bike Stair climbing Elliptic	Boot Brace Shoe/insert	20	4
Week 3	Stationary bike Stair climbing Elliptic	Boot Brace Shoe/insert	30	4

Start the cardiovascular program with the stationary bike. Once you are able to ride the bike 30 minutes per day 4 days per week, you may replace 1 day per week of biking with stair-climbing or elliptic equipment. Exercise on the stair-climbing or elliptic equipment for the same amount of time you would on the stationary bike.

with a stair or incline board for 3 minutes three times per day. Single leg balance is initiated with a regular shoe and then progressed to a bare foot on a hard surface. The initial goal is 60 seconds. Once this is attained, balance can be advanced using a soft surface and balance board. Biking in the boot can be substituted with a progression of elliptic and stair-climbing exercises using a brace and athletic shoe. An independent home exercise program is given to each patient to be performed two to three times per day.[28]

Phase III

Phase III is the final phase of rehabilitation before return to sport. This phase is typically implemented around 2 months after surgery and focuses on advanced strengthening of the entire lower extremity, flexibility, proprioception, and sport-specific agility drills. Once the athlete can use a stair-climbing or elliptic machine for 30 minutes 4 to 5 days a week without difficulty, he or she may transition to running. It is important at this phase to give the athlete a set of running guidelines that allows for gradual progression of activity (**Table 3**). The final goal of phase III is the return to sport after successfully completing a sport-specific functional progression program, including running without discomfort (**Box 1**).[28]

DISCUSSION

There is a spectrum of unstable ankle injuries encountered by the orthopedic surgeon who provides care for athletes, ranging from isolated malleolar fractures to complete syndesmosis disruptions. Each injury pattern should be treated individually, but the overall goal is to allow the athlete to return to sport as quickly and safely as possible. Much has been written about treatment and subsequent rehabilitation in the general population, but there is little in the literature looking at outcomes and prognostic indicators for the athlete. Porter and colleagues[11] were the first to publish a study looking at the prognosis for athletes with surgically reduced and rigidly fixed ankle fractures while providing a timeline for return to sport.

There has been a transition in the general population from prolonged immobilization to functional rehabilitation with early ROM and weight bearing, provided that rigid anatomic fixation is achieved. Preceding studies have demonstrated that integrating early functional motion and weight bearing leads to expedited return to work and activities of daily living.[5,13,35,36]

There are a limited number of studies in the literature investigating unstable ankle injuries in athletes. Donley and colleagues[26] reported on a series of three professional football players with pronation-external rotation injures. All three were able to return to

Table 3
Functional progression running

Week No.	Day							Total minutes
	1	2	3	4	5	6	7	
1	10	0	10	0	12	0	14	36
2	0	16	0	18	0	20	0	54
3	25	20	0	25	25	0	30	125
4	30	0	30	35	0	35	40	170
5	0	40	35	0	45	40	45	215

Previously running 30 to 45 minutes per day.

Box 1
Functional progression: field sports

Begin with step one. If you can do this exercise without pain or limping, you may proceed to the next step. It is very important that you perform each exercise correctly, without apprehension. When you have successfully completed each step of the functional progression, you may then attempt to return to your sport. You should wear a brace or tape if instructed.

Heel raises, injured leg—10 times

Walk at fast pace—50 yards

Jumping on both legs—10 times

Jumping on the injured leg—10 times

Jog straight—50 yards

Jog straight and curves—2 laps

Sprint: one-half, three-quarters, and full speed—40 yards

Run figures of eight: one-half, three-quarters, and full speed—15 yards

Cariocas (cross-overs), 40 yards—both directions

Backward running—40 yards

Cutting: one-half, three-quarters, and full speed

Position drills

---

their preinjury level of play without pain or stiffness. These investigators did not report on time to return to full participation, however. Tropp and Norlin[37] performed a prospective randomized study looking at early mobilization after ankle fracture. Thirty patients were treated with ORIF, and all were able to begin weight bearing immediately. One group was randomized to a plaster cast for 6 weeks, whereas a second group was placed in a brace for early motion after surgery. Impaired muscle torque and ROM limitations were significantly less in the brace group at 10 weeks and 1 year. Fritschy[38] evaluated a group of 10 professional skiers with syndesmotic injuries. Three were treated with operative stabilization, and all were able to return to their previous level of competition. Taylor and colleagues[39] evaluated a group of six male intercollegiate athletes treated with ORIF for a grade III syndesmosis sprain. All were treated with one 4.5-mm, stainless-steel, noncannulated cortical screw. Patients were allowed to begin ROM exercises, progressive weight bearing, and progressive activity as tolerated at 1 week after surgery. Screws were not removed until after the season if the athlete was injured in midseason. The average time to return to full activity was 41 days, and the average Sports Ankle Rating System score was 96.2 at 34 months of follow-up. No complications were noted, but one screw broke during removal and 2 patients had mild degenerative changes on lateral radiographs at final follow-up. Blauth and colleagues[40] reported on 51 patients treated with tibial pilon fractures. Only five of the injuries occurred during sporting activity, and time to return and level of activity were not addressed. Of the patients involved in athletic activity, 59% resumed their former sporting activity, 27% played at a reduced level, and 14% were unable to return at all. Letts and colleagues[41] reported on a series of seven adolescents who sustained pilon fractures. Four of the seven were injured during sporting activity. Of the four sustaining the injury during athletics, three had an excellent result and one had a good result. These investigators did not report length of time to return to sport.

The senior author (DAP) favors standard repair of the deltoid ligament in syndesmosis injuries and bimalleolar equivalent injuries. The literature to date is unclear regarding the standard need for repair. Nevertheless, the authors see three advantages to standard repair of the deltoid ligament for these injuries. First, the joint can be evaluated from the medial side to visualize potential articular chondral or osteochondral lesions. The authors perform a medial arthrotomy first so that they can sublux the ankle to assess the talar dome and distal tibia surfaces. Second, with the proposed aggressive approach to motion and weight bearing without cast immobilization, deltoid repair is a way to mitigate against laxity in the deltoid and potential insufficiency. Finally, there is no reliable reconstructive procedure for an incompetent deltoid ligament, so the authors want to be certain that they have medial stability.

Fixation of the syndesmosis can be quite variable. There are multiple reports in the literature using a spectrum of syndesmosis fixation, including one or two screws with a diameter of 3.5-mm to 4.5-mm crossing three or four cortices. Most orthopedic surgeons use solid screws; however, the senior author (DAP) uses cannulated screws for fixation of the syndesmosis. Advantages of cannulated screw fixation include relative ease of removal in the case of screw fracture. The screw can be removed using the reverse thread extractor within the cannulated screw from the broken screw removal set. This obviates the need to overdrill from the medial or lateral side and to remove more bone, potentially creating a stress riser.[11] Also, insertion of the screw is made easier by first placing the thin guide pin and documenting optimal placement before drilling across the syndesmosis.

It is important for the treating physician to provide a timeline for the athlete's recovery and potential return to competition to the athlete, coaches, and athletic trainer. Porter and colleagues[11] were able to provide a timeline in their review of athletes treated for unstable ankle injuries. Athletes with isolated lateral malleolar fractures were the earliest to return to athletic competition. This finding was likely attributable to the lower energy of injury and relative ease of fibular reduction. Bimalleolar fractures and syndesmosis disruptions were similar in their time frame for return to full participation. Syndesmosis injuries required removal of the syndesmosis screws, typically at 12 weeks, before release to athletic competition. Adolescent athletes with Salter-Harris type fractures had a similar return to sport compared with athletes with isolated lateral malleolar fractures.[11]

Athletes treated with rigid anatomic fixation followed by a rehabilitation program consisting of early ROM and weight bearing can safely return to sport 1 to 4 months after surgery, depending on the specific injury pattern. The intent of an accelerated rehabilitation program is to incorporate the normal fracture and soft tissue healing with ROM and strengthening so that the athlete can attain a rapid and complete recovery.

SUMMARY

Athletes with unstable ankle injuries treated with rigid and anatomic internal fixation with concomitant repair of indicated ligaments followed by an accelerated rehabilitation program consisting of early weight bearing and near-immediate ROM can obtain excellent outcomes. Early ROM and weight bearing, if indicated depending on the specific injury pattern, can be effective with low morbidity. Return to sports can be expected as early as 4 weeks after rigid fixation of an isolated fibula fracture and up to 8 to 10 weeks after stabilization of a bimalleolar equivalent fracture with deltoid repair. Syndesmosis fixation can take up to 4 to 6 months before successful return to sport.

REFERENCES

1. Carr JB. Malleolar fractures and soft tissue injuries of the ankle. In: Browner BD, Jupiter JB, Levine AM, et al, editors. Skeletal trauma. 3rd edition. Philadelphia: Saunders; 2003. p. 2307–74.
2. MacAuley D. Ankle injuries: same joint, different sports. Med Sci Sports Exerc 1999;31(11 Suppl):S409–11.
3. Garrick JG, Requa RK. The epidemiology of foot and ankle injuries. Clin Sports Med 1988;7(1):29–36.
4. Backx FJ, Erich WB, Kemper AB, et al. Sports injuries in school-aged children. An epidemiologic study. Am J Sports Med 1989;17(2):234–40.
5. Egol KA, Dolan R, Koval KJ. Functional outcome of surgery for fractures of the ankle. A prospective, randomized comparison of management in a cast or a functional brace. J Bone Joint Surg Br 2000;82(2):246–9.
6. Dahners LE. The pathogenesis and treatment of bimalleolar ankle fractures. Instr Course Lect 1990;39:85–94.
7. Lindsjö U. Operative treatment of ankle fracture-dislocations. A follow-up study of 306/321 consecutive cases. Clin Orthop Relat Res 1985;199:28–38.
8. Tunturi T, Kemppainen K, Pätiälä H, et al. Importance of anatomical reduction for subjective recovery after ankle fracture. Acta Orthop Scand 1983;54(4):641–7.
9. Yablon IG, Heller FG, Shouse L. The key role of the lateral malleolus in displaced fractures of the ankle. J Bone Joint Surg Am 1977;59(2):169–73.
10. Ramsey PL, Hamilton W. Changes in tibiotalar area of contact caused by lateral talar shift. J Bone Joint Surg Am 1976;58:356–7.
11. Porter DA, May B, Berney T. Functional outcome after operative treatment for distal fibula and tibia fractures in young athletes: a retrospective, case series. Foot Ankle Int 2008;29(9):887–94.
12. Bauer M, Bergström B, Hemborg A, et al. Malleolar fractures: nonoperative versus operative treatment. A controlled study. Clin Orthop Relat Res 1985;199: 17–27.
13. Burwell HN, Charnley AD. The treatment of displaced fractures at the ankle by rigid internal fixation and early joint movement. J Bone Joint Surg Br 1965; 47(4):634–60.
14. Chandler RW. Management of complex ankle fractures in athletes. Clin Sports Med 1988;7(1):127–41.
15. Davis AW, Alexander IJ. Problematic fractures and dislocations in the foot and ankle of athletes. Clin Sports Med 1990;9(1):163–81.
16. Phillips WA, Schwartz HS, Keller CS, et al. A prospective, randomized study of the management of severe ankle fractures. J Bone Joint Surg Am 1985;67(1): 67–78.
17. Roberts RS. Surgical treatment of displaced ankle fractures. Clin Orthop Relat Res 1983;172:164–70.
18. Klossner O. Late results of operative and non-operative treatment of severe ankle fractures. A clinical study. Acta Chir Scand Suppl 1962;293:1–93.
19. Walheim T, Akerman N. Intraarticular malleolar fractures. Acta Chir Scand 1936; 79:166.
20. Segal D, Wiss DA, Whitelaw GP. Functional bracing and rehabilitation of ankle fractures. Clin Orthop Relat Res 1985;199:39–45.
21. Inman VT. The joints of the ankle. Baltimore (MD): Williams & Wilkins; 1976.
22. Earll M, Wayne J, Brodrick C, et al. Contribution of the deltoid ligament to ankle joint characteristics: a cadaver study. Foot Ankle Int 1996;17:317–24.

23. Walling AK, Sanders RW. Ankle fractures. In: Coughlin MJ, Mann RA, Saltzman CL, editors. Surgery of the foot and ankle. 8th edition. Philadelphia: Mosby Elsevier; 2007. p. 1973–2016.

24. Maisonneuve JG. Recherches sur la fracture du perone. Arch Med Gen Trop 1840;7:165, 433 [in French].

25. Kay RM, Matthys GA. Pediatric ankle fractures: evaluation and treatment. J Am Acad Orthop Surg 2001;9:268–78.

26. Donley BG, Maschke S, Bergfeld JA, et al. Pronation-external rotation ankle fractures in 3 professional football players. Am J Orthop 2005;34(11):547–50.

27. Cooper PS. Proprioception in injury prevention and rehabilitation of ankle sprains. In: Sammarco GJ, editor. Rehabilitation of the foot and ankle. St Louis (MO): Mosby; 1995: 95–105.

28. Barill ER, Porter DA. Principles of rehabilitation for the foot and ankle. In: Porter DA, Schon LC, editors. Baxter's the foot and ankle in sport. 2nd edition. Philadelphia: Mosby; 2008. p. 595–610.

29. Gelberman RH, Nunley JA, Osterman AL. Influences of the protected passive mobilization interval on flexor tendon healing. A prospective randomized clinical study. Clin Orthop Relat Res 1991;264:189–96.

30. Aoki M, Kubota H, Pruitt DL. Biomechanical and histologic characteristics of canine flexor tendon repair using early postoperative mobilization. J Hand Surg [Am] 1997;22(1):107–14.

31. Duran RJ, et al. Management of flexor tendon lacerations in zone 2 using controlled passive motion postoperatively. In: Hunter JM, et al, editors. Rehabilitation of the hand. St Louis (MO): Mosby; 1978.

32. Shelbourne KD, Nitz P. Accelerated rehabilitation after anterior cruciate ligament reconstruction. Am J Sports Med 1990;18(3):292–9.

33. Salter RB, Simmonds DF, Malcolm BW, et al. The biological effect of continuous passive motion on the healing of full-thickness defects in articular cartilage. An experimental investigation in the rabbit. J Bone Joint Surg Am 1980;62(8): 1232–51.

34. Trappe SW, Trappe TA, Lee GA, et al. Comparison of a space shuttle flight (STS-78) and bed rest on human muscle function. J Appl Phys 2001;91(1):57–64.

35. Lehtonen H, Järvinen TL, Honkonen S, et al. Use of a cast compared with a functional ankle brace after operative treatment of an ankle fracture. A prospective, randomized study. J Bone Joint Surg Am 2003;85(A-2):205–11.

36. Simanski CJ, Maegele MG, Lefering R, et al. Functional treatment and early weightbearing after an ankle fracture: a prospective study. J Orthop Trauma 2006;20(2):108–14.

37. Tropp H, Norlin R. Ankle performance after ankle fracture: a randomized study of early mobilization. Foot Ankle Int 1995;16(2):79–83.

38. Fritschy D. An unusual ankle injury in top skiers. Am J Sports Med 1989;17(2): 282–5.

39. Taylor DC, Tenuta JJ, Uhorchak JM, et al. Aggressive surgical treatment and early return to sports in athletes with grade III syndesmosis sprains. Am J Sports Med 2007;35(11):1833–8.

40. Blauth M, Bastian L, Krettek C, et al. Surgical options for the treatment of severe tibial pilon fractures: a study of three techniques. J Orthop Trauma 2001;15(3): 153–60.

41. Letts M, Davidson D, McCaffrey M. The adolescent pilon fracture: management and outcome. J Pediatr Orthop 2001;21(1):20–6.

Peroneal Tendon Tears, Surgical Management and Its Complications

Rebecca A. Cerrato, MD*, Mark S. Myerson, MD

KEYWORDS

- Peroneal tears • Peroneus brevis • Peroneus longus
- Peroneal instability

Peroneal tendon injuries in the athlete are recognized with increasing frequency as a pathologic entity. Once considered uncommon, they have been attributed to many cases of persistent lateral ankle symptoms after a "typical" ankle sprain. Acute tears of the peroneus brevis, and less commonly the peroneus longus, have been implicated in sport activities and are often coexistent with peroneal instability.[1] Monteggia[2] first described peroneal subluxation in a ballet dancer. Skiers are at particular risk because of the forced dorsiflexion of the ankle that occurs in a rapid stop with deceleration.[3] Subluxation typically occurs in cases in which the foot is in a dorsiflexed position and the peroneal muscles strongly contract, causing an eversion force simultaneously.[4,5] Peroneal instability, as well as tearing, has also been linked to soccer, tennis, American football, running, basketball, and ice-skating.[6–9]

ANATOMY AND BIOMECHANICS

The origin of the peroneus longus muscle is from the proximal fibular head extending to the proximal two thirds of the fibula. The musculotendinous junction ends proximal to the lateral malleolus. The peroneus longus tendon then passes into a fibro-osseous tunnel, in common with the peroneus brevis tendon and behind the lateral malleolus. In the tunnel, the two tendons share a common synovial sheath enveloping them. The tendon then runs below the peroneal tubercle, where the common tendon sheath bifurcates. Both the tendons then pass under the inferior peroneal retinaculum approximately 2 to 3 cm distal to the tip of the fibula.[10] The peroneus longus enters a second tunnel that is created by the long plantar ligament and the peroneal groove of the cuboid. Within this tunnel, the os peroneum, a sesamoid bone present in 10% to 20% of human feet, is located.[11] Its insertion is onto the plantar base of the first metatarsal and the medial cuneiform.

The Institute for Foot and Ankle Reconstruction, Mercy Medical Center, 302 St. Paul Place, Baltimore, MD 21202, USA
* Corresponding author.
E-mail address: boohinck2@yahoo.com (R.A. Cerrato).

Foot Ankle Clin N Am 14 (2009) 299–312
doi:10.1016/j.fcl.2009.01.004
1083-7515/09/$ – see front matter © 2009 Elsevier Inc. All rights reserved.

foot.theclinics.com

The peroneus brevis muscle originates from the lower two thirds of the lateral fibula. It lies medial and anterior to the peroneus longus muscle. The musculotendinous junction for the peroneus brevis ends at the lateral malleolus; however, it can often extend 2 to 3 cm beyond.[12] The broad peroneus brevis tendon lies directly on the retromalleolar groove and is compressed by the peroneus longus tendon. Distal to the tip of the lateral malleolus, it courses over the calcaneofibular ligament and the peroneal tubercle, within its own synovial sheath. It inserts at the base of the fifth metatarsal.

Because the peroneals descend behind the lateral malleolus, they are contained within a fibro-osseous tunnel formed by the fibular groove and the superior peroneal retinaculum (SPR).[13] The fibular groove is jointly derived from the lateral malleolus and its associated periosteum. Similar to the labrum in the shoulder and hip, the postero-lateral aspect of the malleolus has a fibrocartilaginous rim that serves to deepen the fibular groove. The SPR, located 1 cm proximal to the tip of the fibula, originates from this ridge and inserts onto the lateral wall of the calcaneus, with variable other insertions often including the anterior Achilles tendon sheath.[14,15] Differences in the anatomy of the groove may predispose some individuals to peroneal instability. Edwards,[16] examining 178 fibulae, noted that a sulcus was present in the bone in 82% of cases, the bone was flat in 11%, and 7% had convex surfaces. Recently, Ozbag and colleagues[17] performed a cadaver study on 93 fibulae and found that 63 (68%) had a concave groove, whereas a flat or convex area was observed in the remaining specimens.

The blood supply to the peroneal tendons has been described previously in several studies.[18,19] The main blood supply for the peroneal tendons is from the posterior peroneal artery, with branches of the medial tarsal artery supplying the distal part of the peroneus longus. The blood vessels enter the highly vascularized peritenon through separate vincula from the posterolateral aspect of both tendons. The vessels then penetrate the tendon tissue and anastomose with an intratendinous arterial network. Peterson and colleagues[18] studied the peroneal blood supply using injections and immunohistochemical methods in cadaver specimens and found three distinct avascular zones within the tendons. The intratendinous blood supply of the peroneus brevis tendon is interrupted at the fibular groove. The peroneus longus tendon had two avascular zones: (1) the region where the tendon turns around the lateral malleolus and the peroneal tubercle, and (2) the region where the tendon changes direction under the cuboid. As with other tendons with watershed zones, they are susceptible to chronic degenerative changes.

An accessory muscle in the lateral compartment of the leg, the peroneus quartus, can also be present (**Fig. 1**). Its incidence as reported in the literature ranges from 6.6%[20] to 21.7%.[21] It can have varying anatomic characteristics with respect to its origin and insertion, but it most commonly originates from fibers of the peroneus brevis and inserts onto the peroneal tubercle of the calcaneus. It has been associated with peroneal tendinopathy, including brevis tears, instability, and stenosing tenosynovitis. The tendon causes symptoms by virtue of the bulk behind the fibula contained by the retinaculum. It is difficult to make the diagnosis of this preoperatively, even using MRI images, because the accessory tendon and muscle appears like a split in the peroneus brevis.

The peroneus longus functions as the primary evertor of the foot, first metatarsal plantarflexor, and secondary ankle plantarflexor. The peroneus brevis acts to evert and abduct the foot and as a secondary ankle plantarflexor.[22] The peroneus longus contributes 35% and the peroneus brevis 28% of hindfoot eversion power.[23] They serve as dynamic stabilizers for the ankle and hindfoot against inversion forces.

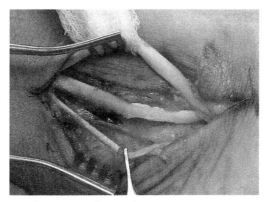

Fig. 1. Peroneus qaurtus demonstrated using forceps.

MECHANISM OF INJURY
Peroneal Tendon Instability

Acute peroneal tendon dislocations most commonly result from a sudden, forceful, passive dorsiflexion of an everted foot with a sudden, strong contraction of the peroneal muscles.[3] However, this injury has also been described with the foot in inversion, again with a sudden contraction of the peroneals.[24] The vigorous contraction of the peroneal muscles causes the retinaculum to tear or strip off the fibula at its periosteal attachment. The peroneus brevis dislocates to the front of the fibula, and although the longus can follow the brevis, it typically does not pass in front of the distal fibula with dislocation.[24] Peroneal tendon subluxation is commonly associated with tears of the brevis, particularly if ankle instability is present.[15,25–28] In a cadaver study, Geppert and colleagues[15] described parallel alignment of the SPR and the calcaneofibular ligament, noting that the SPR acts as a secondary restraint to ankle inversion and that disruption of the lateral collateral ankle ligaments places significant strain on the SPR. This has particular clinical significance because the peroneals must be carefully examined in cases in which chronic ankle instability is present.

Peroneus Brevis Tears

The true incidence of peroneus brevis tears is unknown. Two cadaveric studies performed by Sobel and colleagues[29,30] reported varying incidences of such tears, from 11.3% to 37%, in elderly patients. The tears are typically longitudinal and generally from 2.5 to 5.0 cm in length.[12] Several mechanisms have been implicated by etiologic study of peroneus brevis tears. The position of the peroneus brevis in the peroneal tunnel allows for repetitive compressive loads of the peroneus longus over the flattened brevis in the retromalleolar groove.[31] Subluxation of the peroneus brevis with injury of the tendon as it passes over the sharp posterolateral edge of the fibula, creating a buttonhole defect, has been maintained to be a primary cause of peroneus brevis tears.[32,33] An incompetent SPR is frequently found in patients who have peroneus brevis tears, and the authors and other investigators have noted that repetitive ankle inversion sprains, chronic lateral ankle instability, and generalized ligamentous laxity are causes of SPR laxity.[34] Investigators have stated that a shallow fibular groove may predispose a patient to the tendon instability.[16,17] However, this is debatable. Although a flattened groove has been hypothesized as one of the predisposing causes of peroneal tendon subluxation, the evidence is mostly anecdotal, and the hypothesis has not been proven prospectively, Even if one notes a flattened groove on a CT image or operatively in patients who have recurrent and chronic dislocation of the tendons, one cannot prove that the shallowness of the groove was the causative agent. Although the groove has been demonstrated anatomically to be convex or concave in a certain percentage of patients, the continued pressure of the peroneal tendons behind the fibula is required to maintain the shape of the groove. The authors have noted a similar problem in patients who have a chronic dislocation of the posterior tibial tendon, in whom at surgery a flat or absent groove was present; yet for each of the patients in this study, there was a definite cause of the dislocation that was not related to the shape of the medial malleolus.[35] The authors have noted the same problem with the peroneal tendons after trauma, particularly after acute calcaneus fractures. The peroneal tendons are commonly injured or subluxated or the retinaculum is torn in acute calcaneus fractures, and if not repaired, the tendons remain chronically dislocated. During subsequent reconstruction in these patients, the authors noted that the groove was absent as early as 9 months after the initial fracture occurred, again indicating that the pressure from the peroneal tendons on the fibula is necessary to maintain the surface contour of the groove.[36] Finally, other investigators have stated that stenosis within the peroneal tunnel as the result of the presence of an anomalous, low-lying brevis muscle belly[37,38] or the presence of a peroneus quartus [20,21] can result in SPR laxity and increased strains directly on the brevis tendon.

Peroneus Longus Tears

Tears of the peroneus longus are much less common, but may coexist with ruptures of the brevis. Ruptures occur at the tip of the lateral malleolus, peroneal tubercle, or os peroneum.[11,39–41] As with the peroneus brevis, injury to the peroneus longus can be acute or chronic. Chronic injury to the peroneus longus is attributable to tendon degeneration with longitudinal splitting, which is often seen in patients participating in athletics after a period of inactivity.[31] An acute injury to a healthy tendon typically is a result of a sudden inversion sprain or forced eversion of a supinated foot. In the presence of an os peroneum, the tendon rupture is caused by an avulsion fracture with diastasis and proximal retraction of the tendon or the sesamoid itself (**Fig. 2**).[11] Not having an os present does not rule out a peroneus longus injury. A hypertrophied peroneal tubercle subjects the peroneus longus to abnormal shear stresses and is associated with attrition of this tendon.[41] One of the more common causes of tears of the longus tendon is associated with a varus deformity of the heel or a cavovarus foot deformity. The varus position of the heel increases the force not only on the peroneals, but on the peroneal tubercle hypertrophies as well. The authors have noted this condition in numerous athletes, finding that the pathologic conditions range from stenosis of the tendons to splits and longitudinal tears of one or both tendons (**Fig. 3**).

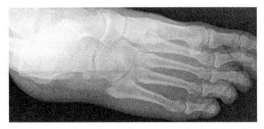

Fig. 2. Oblique foot radiograph of the foot of a 22-year-old basketball player who sustained an inversion ankle injury. He complained of severe lateral foot pain. The radiograph reveals the os peroneum retracted proximally.

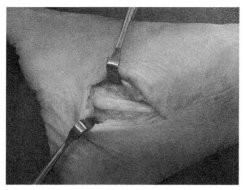

Fig. 3. An intraoperative example of a hypertrophied peroneal tubercle, with thickening and degeneration of the peroneus longus secondary to chronic stenosis and shearing.

PATIENT EVALUATION

Symptoms may be subtle, particularly in patients who have partial tears, and can often be misdiagnosed. Frequently, a patient will report a history of an ankle sprain that has not resolved. Always evaluate the patient who has chronic ankle instability for pain behind the lateral malleolus and the lateral side of foot.

Clinical Findings

On examination, swelling over the peroneal tendons is the most consistent finding in patients who have partial tears. Palpation along the course of both peroneal tendons may elicit tenderness or thickness over the location of a chronic tear or diffusely in the presence of an acute injury. Peroneus longus ruptures often are tender at the cuboid groove. Pain can be reproduced using resisted hindfoot eversion and ankle dorsiflexion or using passive hindfoot inversion and ankle plantarflexion. Unless the tears are chronic, power of eversion, although painful, is typically present and ankle motion is preserved. During ankle motion evaluation, palpation over the tendon sheath can reveal crepitus, clicking, or snapping. Raikin and colleagues[42] described a subgroup of patients who had intrasheath subluxation of the peroneal tendons within the fibular groove with intact SPRs. When examined using circumduction of the ankle, particularly at the phase of maximum eversion and dorsiflexion, these patients demonstrated a palpable and often painful click. However, the peroneal tendons remained behind the fibula. Using dynamic ultrasonography, the investigators identified the peroneus brevis and longus tendons subluxing over one another within the peroneal groove.

Hindfoot and forefoot alignment is evaluated with the patient standing. If hindfoot varus is present, a Coleman block test should be performed to determine if the hindfoot varus is the primary problem or secondary to a plantarflexed first ray seen in patients who have cavovarus feet. Have the patient perform both single- and double-heel rise while standing to assess stability and balance, and always check for ankle instability. Peroneal tendon subluxation can be reproduced using active resisted eversion of the ankle or circumduction of the foot. The ankle can also be actively dorsiflexed and plantarflexed while being everted against resistance. Most patients who have chronic pathologic conditions will be apprehensive as the tendon perches on the edge of the fibula about to subluxate. Patients with an acute subluxation demonstrate substantial swelling, tenderness, and ecchymosis behind the distal fibula, and provocative maneuvers are not typically helpful because of pain.

Imaging

Weight-bearing radiographs of the foot and ankle should be obtained when evaluating for peroneal pathology. Document the alignment and the presence of an os peroneum, hypertrophied peroneal tubercle, and arthrosis. Foot radiographs may reveal a fracture of the fifth metatarsal base, which clinically may mimic a peroneus brevis tear. Ankle radiographs may reveal a "fleck sign," which is a small avulsion fracture of the lateral malleolus (**Fig. 4**).[27] This finding is pathognomonic for an acute dislocation of the peroneal tendons.

Ultrasound imaging has been employed in diagnosing peroneal tendon tears. It is noninvasive, inexpensive, and does not expose the patient to radiation. Dynamic real-time ultrasonography is used to examine the tendons throughout their physiologic range of motion. The gliding motion of the peroneal tendons within their sheaths may help differentiate tenosynovitis from tendon injuries.[40] Furthermore, it allows the radiologist to perform provocative maneuvers to identify peroneal subluxation. Ultrasound imaging can help radiologists distinguish between the presence of peritendinous fluid, tendinosis, and partial or complete tears. Grant and colleagues[40] reported the sensitivity, specificity, and accuracy of ultrasonography when used in diagnosing peroneal tears at 100%, 85%, and 90%, respectively. The biggest limitation to this modality is that it is operator-dependent, with a variable learning curve.

MRI has become the standard imaging modality for peroneal tendon disorders. Torn tendons typically appear thickened, display increased intrasubstance signal intensity on T1- and T2-weighted images, and have irregular contours. Areas of increased signal intensity are best studied using oblique axial images.[12] A peroneus brevis tear can appear to be C-shaped or bisected (**Fig. 5**).[43] Peroneus longus tears may reveal linear or round areas of increased signal intensity. Steel and DeOrio[44] reported the specificity of MRI to be 80% in detecting peroneus brevis tears, 100% for peroneus longus tears, and 60% for the detection of tears in both tendons. However, MRI findings can be unreliable, with false-positive and false-negative results reported.[12,26,45] Increased signal intensity can be a result of the magic-angle phenomenon. On T1-weighted images, signal intensity increased in cases in which the tendon was at a 55° angle to the axis of the magnetic field. Because this effect is not present when using long echo times, the absence of abnormal signal intensity on T2-weighted

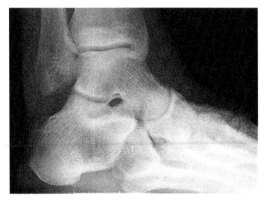

Fig. 4. A mortise ankle radiograph that reveals an avulsion fracture off the posterolateral fibula, diagnostic of an acute injury to the peroneal retinaculum, which is usually associated with subluxation or dislocation of the tendons.

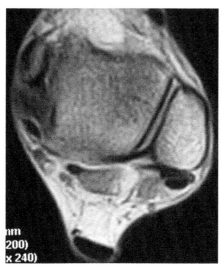

Fig. 5. A T1-weighted axial image that shows irregularity of the peroneus brevis with increased intrasubstance signal intensity.

images suggests an intact tendon. Therefore, a diagnosis of peroneal tendon tears should rely on the patient's history and the clinical exam. MRI performed with the foot placed in marked plantarflexion minimizes the magic-angle effect on ankle tendons.[12]

MANAGEMENT

When an athlete is symptomatic because of a tear, subluxation, or dislocation, is surgery necessary? Put differently, will the tear become more significant if surgery is not performed? Certainly, tenosynovitis or irritation of the tendons caused by a mechanical abnormality can be treated nonoperatively using appropriate therapies, as noted later in this article. If the symptoms are minor, tolerated by the athlete, and diminished with treatment, then surgery can be delayed or may not be necessary. Treatment of a tendon tear or dislocation is by and large done using surgery. Conservative therapy includes the use of nonsteroidal anti-inflammatory medication, a lateral heel wedge, physical therapy, and immobilization in a short-leg walking cast or boot. In the presence of peroneal instability, the results of nonoperative treatment are less encouraging.[3] Although nonoperative treatment of an acute peroneal tendon dislocation has been described,[10] the authors would not recommend it in the athlete.

Operative management of peroneal tendon tears is dictated by the location and severity of the pathology. Sobel and colleagues[34] described four grades of peroneus brevis tears to help guide their management of the injuries (**Table 1**). Krause and Brodsky[33] stated that the cross-sectional area of the tendon affected is more important with regard to prognosis and treatment than its length. They classify peroneus brevis lesions as Grade I if there is less than 50% tendon involvement and Grade II if there is greater than 50%, and they recommend repair for Grade I lesions only. The authors, however, note that this is arbitrary, because the tendon usually splits into two parts, one occasionally being thicker than the other. A repair should always be attempted in the athlete, even if there are multiple splits present.

Table 1	
Classification system of peroneus brevis tears	
Grade	Description
I	Splaying of the tendon
II	Partial thickness split <1 cm in diameter
III	Full thickness split 1–2 cm in diameter
IV	Full thickness split >2 cm in diameter

(*From* Sobel M, Geppert MJ, Olson EJ, Bohne, WH, et al. The dynamics of peroneus brevis tendon splits: A proposed mechanism, technique of diagnosis, and classification of injury. Foot Ankle Int 1992;13:413–22; with permission. Copyright © 1992 by the American Orthopedic Foot and Ankle Society, Inc.)

Peroneus Brevis Tear

Inspection of the peroneal tendons at the time of surgery should also include evaluation for laxity of the peroneal retinaculum, for the presence of a low-lying brevis muscle belly or peroneus quartus, and for any osteophytes of the fibular groove. An inflamed synovitis is a good indicator of a tendon rupture, and if so, it should be debrided. After being identified, the tear is debrided of fibrous, disorganized, or fatty tissue. Longitudinal, or "buttonhole," tears with splaying and minimal degeneration are repaired into a tubular shape using a running absorbable suture. If the tear is complete and longitudinal, one part of the tendon can be excised and the remaining viable portion repaired. The authors use a running 4.0 suture that is absorbable. A similar suture repair can be used if there is a longitudinal split in the tendon, without excising a strip of the tendon. This gets a little more complicated in cases in which there are multiple splits in the tendon, particularly if they are associated with degeneration. In the athlete, the authors attempt to resect the degenerated portion, preserving viable tendon, which is repaired using a running absorbable suture (**Fig. 6**A, B). If the tendon is not reparable, then a tenodesis to the adjacent remaining peroneus longus tendon can be considered, although the result may not be as predictable as it would be when performing a repair. Squires and colleagues[46] recommend that the tenodesis be performed proximally at least 3 to 4 cm above the tip of the lateral malleolus and distally at least 5 cm below the tip of the lateral malleolus to avoid fibular impingement. Chronic degenerative tears of the peroneus brevis at its insertion may require debridement of the tendon and repair to the fifth metatarsal, with suture anchors or tenodesis to the longus tendon. The authors have treated athletes who had insertional tendinopathy after having fractures of the base of the fifth metatarsal that remained painful using this same approach.

Peroneus Longus Tear

With longitudinal tears of the peroneus longus, surgical principles of tendon repair similar to those outlined previously in this article apply. If the peroneal tubercle is enlarged, it should always be excised. A complete rupture typically occurs at the cuboid tunnel, and if an os peroneum is present, a rupture occurs just distal to or through it. If the os peroneum is present and fractured, excision of the bone with end-to-end repair is attempted. This is not easy, because the os lies under the cuboid and visualization is usually incomplete. If repair of the tendon is attempted, a more extensile incision laterally is required to facilitate exposure of the retracted tendon. An end-to-end repair is not always possible, either because of degeneration of the tendon or an inability to get the tendon ends apposed. In such cases, one can consider a tenodesis of the two tendons or insertion of the longus into the cuboid. Often, the longus tendon requires some debridement, after which it can be transferred to the

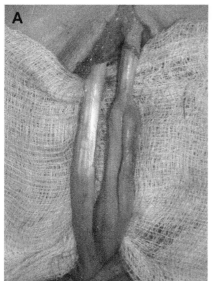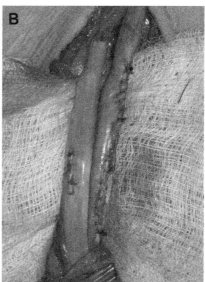

Fig. 6. (*A, B*) Photos from an intraoperative evaluation that revealed a longitudinal tear in the peroneus brevis with greater than 50% of the tendon viable after debridement; therefore, a primary repair using a running absorbable suture was performed.

peroneus brevis[22] or the lateral border of the cuboid.[46] (**Fig. 7**A, B). The authors have some concerns about a transfer of the longus tendon into the brevis in the case of an irreparable longus tendon in the athlete. The side-to-side tenodesis can be associated with chronic scarring, which then may lead to dysfunction or even tearing of the distal stump. If the longus tendon is irreparable and degeneration extends to the tip of the fibula, then a tenodesis must be considered more proximally. Redfern and Myerson[45] recommend basing this decision on the tendon excursion to avoid locking up a functional peroneus brevis to a scarred, fibrotic, and dysfunctional peroneus longus.

Combined Tears

Concomitant tears of both peroneal tendons have rarely been reported in the literature.[31,45] Redfern and Myerson[45] created an algorithm for operative management of peroneal tendon tears based on the operative pathologic conditions (**Table 2**). They emphasized the importance of residual tendon function, excursion of the remaining peroneal musculature, ankle stability, and heel alignment.

Treatment of Associated Pathology

Any deformity of the ankle or hindfoot that could lead to recurrent peroneal tendon injury should be corrected simultaneously with surgery. Ankle instability ideally should be determined preoperatively using stress radiographs, but can certainly be identified and repaired intraoperatively. In the athlete, it is ideal to perform an anatomic reconstruction of the ankle instability, either using a Brostrum procedure or one of the hamstring procedures (allogenic or autogenic) that have been described.[47–49] If the peroneus brevis tendon is torn, then either a repair can be done in combination with a Brostrom procedure or the split anterior portion of the tendon can be used to perform either a modified Chrisman-Snook procedure[40] or an Evans procedure.[50] Sobel and Geppert[51] described performing both using a posteriorly modified Brostrom

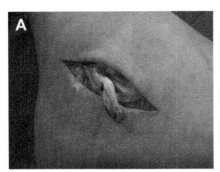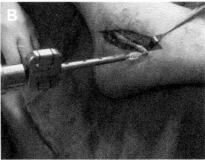

Fig. 7. (A, B) Photos show complete rupture of the peroneus longus at the cuboid tunnel, which required insertion into the cuboid using an interference screw.

Gould procedure. Peroneal tendon instability can be corrected using a fibular groove–deepening procedure and repair of the torn or redundant SPR.

In which cases should hindfoot varus be corrected? Is the calcaneal osteotomy corrective or protective of the repair? If the heel is in varus and associated with a peroneal tear, then it should be corrected. The varus can either be primary, in which case it is usually bilateral, or secondary to the chronic ruptures, in which case the deformity is usually unilateral. Certainly in the latter condition, an osteotomy should be performed and is both corrective and also protective of the repair. The shape and the shift of the osteotomy are determined according to the extent of the heel varus and the calcaneal pitch angle. The authors usually perform a closing-wedge, biplanar, calcaneal osteotomy through the same incision as that used for the peroneal tendon repair. The wedge, of about 6 mm, is removed, and the calcaneus translated slightly laterally. If the pitch angle is increased, then the osteotomy can be simultaneously shifted cephalad.

The addition of a first-metatarsal, dorsal, closing-wedge osteotomy is included in cases of fixed forefoot pronation, which is often observed after a calcaneal osteotomy has been used to correct the hindfoot varus. Chronic overpull of the peroneus longus

Table 2 Algorithm for peroneal tendon surgery	
Intra-Operative Assessment of Peroneal Tendons	
Type I Both tendons grossly intact	Tendon(s) repaired Longitudinal split excised Tendon tubularised
Type II One tendon torn, other 'usable'	Tenodesis performed
Type III Both tendons torn/'unusable'	
Type IIIa No excursion of proximal muscle	Tendon graft (allograft) unlikely to work Tendon transfer performed
Type IIIb Excursion of proximal muscle	If tissue bed scarred then consider staged allograft with silicone rod If no tissue bed scarring then one-stage allograft or tendon transfer performed

creates a gradual, rigid, plantarflexed first metatarsal, which is widely recognized as a dynamic factor causing hindfoot varus and lateral ankle instability.[52] Similar to the calcaneal osteotomy, the shift and size of the wedge is determined based on the extent of first metatarsal plantarflexion and adduction.

OUTCOMES

Reports on the outcomes of the surgical management of peroneal tendon tears are either retrospective reviews or case reviews, and therefore it is difficult to recommend one treatment or another based on these reports. Bassett and Speer[32] retrospectively reviewed the cases of eight collegiate-level athletes treated using primary repair of peroneal tendon tears. They reported that all of the athletes returned to full athletic activity and were asymptomatic, however no validated clinical assessment tool was used in reaching these conclusions. Krause and Brodsky[33] reported on 20 patients treated surgically for peroneus brevis tendon tears. The average postoperative American Orthopaedic Foot and Ankle Society (AOFAS) score was 85. In their discussion, they point out that although the majority of their patients reported good to excellent results, the time it took for maximum function to return was prolonged. Redfern and Myerson[45] retrospectively evaluated 28 patients followed for a mean of 4.6 years after their peroneal surgery. The average postoperative AOFAS score was 82, and 91% had normal to moderate peroneal strength. Steel and DeOrio[44] more recently reported that only 46% of 30 patients treated surgically for peroneal tendon tears were able to successfully return to athletics.

COMPLICATIONS

Failure to make the proper diagnosis is one of the most common reasons for treatment failure in the patient who has lateral ankle pain. A comprehensive, differential diagnosis should be evaluated for each patient. After the correct diagnosis has been made and surgical intervention has been considered, several problems related to peroneal tendon surgery can decrease the probability of a good outcome. Failure to address hindfoot varus malalignment can lead to recurrent peroneal tendon tearing and ankle instability. As discussed earlier in this article, persistent lateral ankle instability can result in laxity of a repaired SPR and strain on the peroneal tendons.[15,25–28] Complete exposure and inspection of the peroneal tendons will help to avoid missing a tear or an associated pathologic condition, such as a low-lying peroneus brevis muscle belly, peroneus quartus, osteophytes, or hypertrophied peroneal tubercle.

Attempts to repair a tendon using significant degenerative changes and revision repair are usually unsuccessful.[10,33] Common pitfalls associated with performing a tenodesis include suturing a scarred, nonfunctional tendon to its adjacent tendon, rendering both ineffective, and performing the tenodesis too close to the fibular groove, resulting in stenosis or subluxation.[10,46]

REFERENCES

1. Clanton TO, Schon LC. Athletic injuries to the soft tissues of the foot and ankle. In: Mann RA, Coughlin MJ, editors. Surgery of the foot and ankle. St Louis (MO): Mosby; 1993;6(2):1167–1177.
2. Monteggia GB. Instituzini chirurgiche, part III. Milan (Italy): Pirotta E Maspero; 1803. p. 336–41.
3. Oden RR. Tendon injuries about the ankle resulting from skiing. Clin Orthop Relat Res 1987;216:63–9.

4. Zoellner G, Clancy W. Recurrent dislocation of the peroneal tendon. J Bone Joint Surg Am 1979;61:292–4.
5. Sobel M, Warren RF, Brourman S. Lateral ankle instability associated with dislocation of the peroneal tendons treated by the Chrisman-Snook procedure: a case report and literature review. Am J Sports Med 1990;18:539–43.
6. Ferran NA, Olivia F, Maffulli N. Recurrent subluxation of the peroneal tendons. Sports Med 2006;36:839–46.
7. Kilkelly F, McHale K. Acute rupture of the peroneus longus tendon in a runner: a case report and review of the literature. Foot Ankle Int 1994;15:567–9.
8. Larsen E. Longitudinal rupture of the peroneus brevis tendon. J Bone Joint Surg Br 1987;69:340–1.
9. Wind WM, Rohrbacher BJ. Peroneus longus and brevis rupture in a collegiate athlete. Foot Ankle Int 2001;22:140–3.
10. Molloy R, Tisdel C. Failed treatment of peroneal tendon injuries. Foot Ankle Clin 2003;8:115–29.
11. Sobel M, Pavlov H, Geppert MJ, et al. Painful os peroneum syndrome: a spectrum of conditions responsible for plantar lateral foot pain. Foot Ankle Int 1994;15:112–24.
12. Khoury NJ, El-Khoury G, Saltzman CL, et al. Peroneus longus and brevis tendon tears: MR imaging evaluation. Radiology 1996;200:833–41.
13. Kumai T, Benjamin M. The histological structure of the malleolar groove of the fibula in man: its direct bearing on the displacement of peroneal tendons and their surgical repair. J Anat 2003;203:257–62.
14. Davis WH, Sobel M, Deland J, et al. The superior peroneal retinaculum: an anatomic study. Foot Ankle Int 1994;15(5):271–5.
15. Geppert MJ, Sobel M, Bohne WH. Lateral ankle instability as a cause of superior peroneal retinacular laxity: an anatomic and biomechanical study of cadaveric feet. Foot Ankle Int 1993;14:330–4.
16. Edwards ME. The relation of the peroneal tendons to the fibula, calcaneus, and cuboideum. Am J Anat 1928;42:213–53.
17. Ozbag D, Gumusalam Y, Uzel M, et al. Morphometrical features of the human malleolar groove. Foot Ankle Int 2008;29:77–81.
18. Peterson W, Bobka T, Stein V, et al. Blood supply of the peroneal tendons. Acta Orthop Scand 2000;71:168–74.
19. Sobel M, Geppert MJ, Hannafin J, et al. Microvascular anatomy of the peroneal tendons. Foot Ankle Int 1992;13:469–72.
20. Zammit J, Singh D. The peroneus quartus muscle: anatomy and clinical relevance. J Bone Joint Surg Br 2003;85:1134–7.
21. Sobel M, Levy ME, Bohne WH. Congenital variations of the peroneus quartus: an anatomic study. Foot Ankle Int 1990;11:81–9.
22. Slater HK. Acute peroneal tendon tears. Foot Ankle 2007;12:659–74.
23. Clarke HD, Kitaoka HB, Ehman RL. Peroneal tendon injuries. Foot Ankle Int 1998; 19:280–8.
24. Safran MR, O'Malley MR, Fu FH. Peroneal tendon subluxation in athletes: new exam technique, case reports, and review. Med Sci Sports Exerc 1999;31: S487–92.
25. Bonnin M, Tavernier T, Bouysset M. Split lesions of the peroneus brevis tendon in chronic ankle laxity. Am J Sports Med 1997;25:699–703.
26. DiGiovanni BF, Fraga CJ, Cohen BE, et al. Associated injuries found in chronic lateral ankle instability. Foot Ankle Int 2000;21:809–15.
27. Eckert WR, Davis EA Jr. Acute rupture of the peroneal retinaculum. J Bone Joint Surg Am 1976;58:670–2.

28. Strauss JE, Forsberg JA, Lippert FG. Chronic lateral ankle instability and associated conditions: a rationale for treatment. Foot Ankle Int 2007;28:1041–4.
29. Sobel M, Levy ME, Bohne WH. Longitudinal attrition of the peroneus brevis tendon in the fibular groove: an anatomic study. Foot Ankle Int 1990;11:124–8.
30. Sobel M, DiCarlo EF, Bohne WH, et al. Longitudinal splitting of the peroneus brevis tendon: an anatomic and histologic study of cadaveric material. Foot Ankle Int 1991;12:165–70.
31. Sammarco GJ. Peroneal tendon injuries. Orthop Clin North Am 1994;25:135–45.
32. Bassett FH, Speer KP. Longitudinal rupture of the peroneal tendons. Am J Sports Med 1993;21:354–7.
33. Krause JO, Brodsky JW. Peroneus brevis tears: pathophysiology, surgical reconstruction, and clinical results. Foot Ankle Int 1998;19:271–9.
34. Sobel M, Geppert MJ, Olson EJ, et al. The dynamics of peroneus brevis tendon splits: a proposed mechanism, technique of diagnosis, and classification of injury. Foot Ankle Int 1992;13:413–22.
35. Ouzounian TJ, Myerson MS. Dislocation of the posterior tibial tendon. Foot Ankle Int 1992;13:215–9.
36. Myerson M, Quill GE Jr. Late complications of fractures of the calcaneus. J Bone Joint Surg Am 1993;75A:331–41.
37. Freccero DM, Berkowitz MJ. The relationship between tears of the peroneus brevis tendon and the distal extent of its muscle belly: an MRI study. Foot Ankle Int 2006;27:236–9.
38. Geller J, Lin S, Cordas O, et al. Relationship of a low-lying muscle belly to tears of the peroneus brevis tendon. Am J Orthop 2003;33:541–4.
39. Brandes CB, Smith RW. Characterization of patients with primary peroneus longus tendinopathy: a review of twenty-two cases. Foot Ankle Int 2000;21:462–8.
40. Grant TH, Kelikian AS, Jereb SE, et al. Ultrasound diagnosis of peroneal tendon tears: a surgical correlation. J Bone Joint Surg Am 2005;87:1788–94.
41. Hyer CF, Dawson JM, Philbin TM, et al. The peroneal tubercle: description, classification, and relevance to peroneus longus tendon pathology. Foot Ankle Int 2005;26:947–50.
42. Raikin SM, Elias H, Nazarian LN. Intrasheath subluxation of the peroneal tendons. J Bone Joint Surg Am 2008;90A:992–9.
43. Major NM, Helms CA, Fritz RC, et al. The MR imaging appearance of longitudinal split tears of the peroneus brevis tendon. Foot Ankle Int 2000;21:514–9.
44. Steel MW, DeOrio JK. Peroneal tendon tears: return to sports after operative treatment. Foot Ankle Int 2007;28:49–54.
45. Redfern D, Myerson MS. The management of concomitant tears of the peroneus longus and brevis tendons. Foot Ankle Int 2004;25:695–707.
46. Squires N, Myerson MS, Gamba C. Surgical treatment of peroneal tendon tears. Foot Ankle Clin 2007;12:675–95.
47. Ajis A, Younger AS, Maffulli N. Anatomic repair for chronic lateral ankle instability. Foot Ankle Clin 2006;11:539–45.
48. Coughlin MJ, Schenck RC Jr. Lateral ankle reconstruction. Foot Ankle Int 2001; 22:256–8.
49. Espinosa N, Smereck J, Kadakia AR, et al. Operative management of ankle instability: reconstruction with open and percutaneous methods. Foot Ankle Clin 2006; 11:547–65.
50. Girard P, Anderson RB, Davis WH, et al. Clinical evaluation of the modified Brostrom-Evans procedure to restore ankle instability. Foot Ankle Int 1999;20: 246–52.

51. Sobel M, Geppert MJ. Repair of concomitant lateral ankle ligament instability and peroneus brevis splits through a posteriorly modified Brostrom Gould. Foot Ankle 1992;13:224–5.

52. Vienne P, Schoniger R, Helmy N, et al. Hindfoot instability in cavovarus deformity: static and dynamic balancing. Foot Ankle Int 2007;28:96–102.

Surgical Advancements: Arthroscopic Alternatives to Open Procedures: Great Toe, Subtalar Joint, Haglund's Deformity, and Tendoscopy

Carol Frey, MD

KEYWORDS

- Arthroscopy • Great toe • Subtalar joint
- Haglund's deformity • Tendoscopy

This article describes advancements in techniques that can be used for common foot, ankle, and tendon issues in the athlete. Great toe arthroscopy can be an effective treatment for several ailments, and is especially useful for debridement of spurs in association with hallux rigidus. Subtalar and posterior ankle arthroscopy can be very advantageous for chronic subtalar pain and fibrosis and for posterior ankle impingement and posterior debridement of OCLs and scar tissue. Tendonoscopy is a newer means of assessing and treating both peroneal and posterior tibial tendon synovitis and small tears. We discuss diagnostic and technique points in relation to these advanced uses of the arthroscope in the athlete.

GREAT TOE ARTHROSCOPY
Indications

Indications for great toe arthroscopy include osteophytes, hallux rigidus, chondromalacia, osteochondral lesions, loose bodies, arthrofibrosis, synovitis secondary to hyperextension and hyperflexion injuries to the great toe. Diagnostic arthroscopy may be indicated in cases of recurrent swelling, locking, persistent pain, and stiffness

Orthopedic Foot and Ankle Surgery, Orthopedic Surgery, UCLA, 1200 Rosecrans Avenue, Suite 208, Manhattan Beach, CA 90266, USA
E-mail address: footfreymd@aol.com

Foot Ankle Clin N Am 14 (2009) 313–339
doi:10.1016/j.fcl.2009.03.001
1083-7515/09/$ – see front matter © 2009 Elsevier Inc. All rights reserved.

that are recalcitrant to a full regimen of conservative treatment. Arthrodesis of the great toe is also possible with arthroscopic technique. Arthroscopy of the great toe is a relatively new application and therefore indications are still developing and few long-term clinical studies have been published.

Anatomy

Minimal stability is provided by the shallow ball-and-socket articulation between the proximal phalanx (PP) and the metatarsal (MT) head. Soft tissues, including the capsule, ligaments, muscles, and tendons provide most of the support to the first metatarsal phalangeal joint (MTP). The extensor hallucis longus tendon divides the dorsum of the first MTP in half (**Fig. 1**).

The branches of the deep peroneal nerve innervate the lateral half and the branches of the superficial peroneal nerve innervate the medial half of the joint. The terminal branches of the saphenous nerve innervate the medial aspect of the great toe.

On the plantar aspect of the first MTP, the sesamoids are within the medial and the lateral portions of the flexor hallucis brevis (FHB) tendon. The sesamoids are surrounded by the split tendon of the FHB, which sends fibers to the plantar plate and subsequently attaches to the proximal aspect of the proximal phalanx. The plantar plate is a strong fibrous structure that inserts on either side of the MTP joint. The flexor

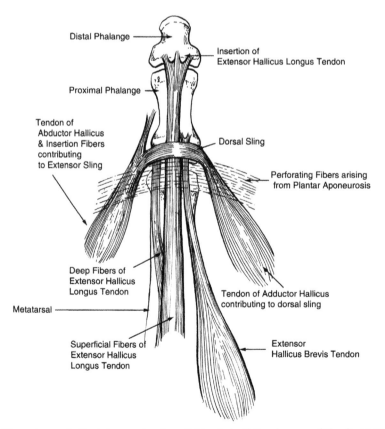

Fig. 1. The extensor hallucis longus tendon divides in half the dorsum of the first MTP.

hallucis longus tendon is both superficial and between the two heads of the FHB tendon.

Biomechanically, the instant center of motion of the first MTP is within the first metatarsal head. Motion occurs between the MT head and the PP by sliding action at the joint surface. In full extension or flexion, this sliding action gives way to compression of the dorsal or plantar articular surfaces of the MT head and PP.

Preoperative Examination

The physical examination of the great toe and sesamoid complex should include range of motion, palpation for points of tenderness and pain, swelling, crepitus, and presence of osteophytes.

The preoperative examination should include a standard standing radiograph of the foot in order to check for osteophytes, osteochondral lesions, joint space narrowing, sesamoid fractures, and other bone pathology (**Fig. 2**).

An MRI may be ordered to evaluate cartilage pathology, osteochondral lesions, sesamoid lesions, and when there is continued pain around the great toe and sesamoid complex in a patient presenting with normal radiographs (**Fig. 3**).

Treatment Options

Nonoperative treatment includes: antiinflammatory medications, a stable shoe or rocker sole shoe, an orthotic device with a sesamoid pad or a Morton's extension, and stretching of the Achilles tendon. When conservative treatment fails, arthroscopic surgery of the great toe is an option.

Instrumentation

- Straight mosquito clamp
- No. 11 blade
- 20-cm3 syringe
- 18-gauge spinal needle
- CHIP [Micro CHIP]
- CHP camera with compatible light source
- Video/TV monitor
- 1.9-, 2.2-, or 2.7-mm oblique, wide-angle 30-degree video arthroscope
- 2.0-mm instrumentation: baskets, grasper, probe, curette
- Sterile toe trap
- Coban to hold toe in toe trap
- Shoulder holder or IV stand to suspend toe traction

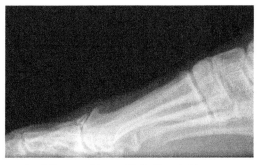

Fig. 2. Lateral radiograph of the great toe with hallux rigidus.

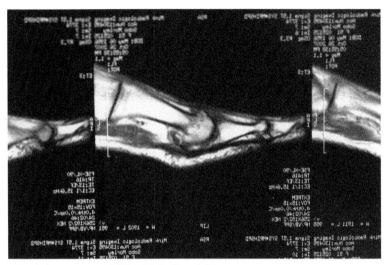

Fig. 3. MRI of the great toe MTP with hallux rigidus.

- 7- to 15-lb sandbag
- Small hand drill
- K-wires
- Tourniquet
- Small radiofrequency wand

Positioning

The patient is placed supine on the operating room table. General, spinal, epidural, or local anesthesia can be used. A sterile finger trap is placed on the toe to suspend the lower extremity, with traction applied at the level of the ankle, if necessary (**Fig. 4**).

Technique

The dorsal medial and dorsal lateral portals are established first (**Fig. 5**). This is accomplished by palpating the joint line just medial or lateral to the extensor hallucis longus tendon. An 18-gauge spinal needle is used to inflate the MTP joint with 5 ml of normal saline. Then a 4-mm longitudinal incision is made for the portal. The subcutaneous tissue is spread with a mosquito clamp to prevent neurovascular injury, and the joint is entered with an interchangeable cannula with semiblunt trochar.

Once visualization of the joint is accomplished through the initial portal, the remaining two portals can be established with a spinal needle under direct vision.

Intraarticular examination includes visualization of 10 major areas (**Fig. 6**):

- Lateral gutter
- Lateral corner of the MT head
- Central portion of the MT head
- Medial corner of the MT head
- Medial gutter
- Medial portion of the PP
- Central portion of the PP
- Lateral portion of the PP
- Medial sesamoid
- Lateral sesamoid

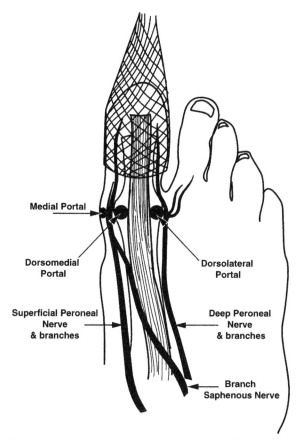

Medial Portal

Dorsomedial Portal

Dorsolateral Portal

Superficial Peroneal Nerve & branches

Deep Peroneal Nerve & branches

Branch Saphenous Nerve

Fig. 4. Position of the patient for great toe arthroscopy using finger trap.

Use of the interchangeable cannula allows rotation of the video arthroscope and instrumentation so that the entire joint and its pathology can be fully evaluated and treated. The 10-point arthroscopic examination is performed through the dorsal lateral portal. The dorsal medial portal provides superior visualization of the dorsal aspect of the metatarsal head and proximal phalanx. The medial and lateral sesamoid are well visualized from the medial portal.

At the conclusion of the arthroscopy, the small portals are closed with 4-0 interrupted nylon sutures. To prevent fistula formation, a bulky compression dressing is applied for 4–7 days.

Technical Tips

Hallux rigidus

The most common indications for arthroscopy of the great toe include treatment of hallux rigidus with a dorsal osteophyte and chondromalacia. Dorsal osteophytes may be removed if they are mild-to-moderate in size. If the osteophyte is large, an open cheilectomy is recommended. The best placement of instruments for an arthroscopic cheilectomy is to place the arthroscope in the dorsal lateral portal, and the

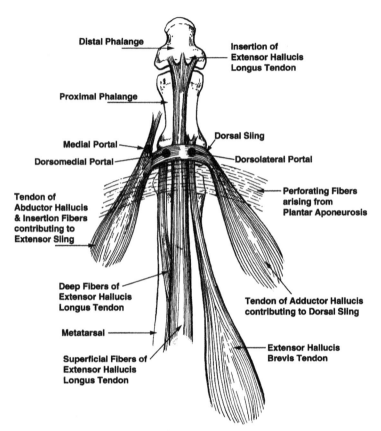

Fig. 5. Portal placement for great toe arthroscopy.

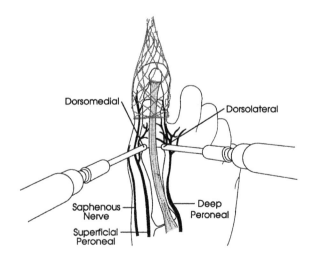

Fig. 6. Examination of the great toe using arthroscopy.

shaver and burr in the dorsomedial or medial portal. Remove the osteophyte from distal to proximal and medial to lateral. When performing an arthroscopic cheilectomy, up to one third of the articular surface may be removed with this technique. However, when performing an arthroscopic cheilectomy, it usually is not necessary to remove as much bone as with an open procedure.

The finger trap is removed before removal of the osteophytes because traction may cause the capsule to pull tight against the osteophyte.

Sesamoid examination

For evaluation and surgery of the medial sesamoid, the dorsolateral portal is used for the arthroscope and the instruments are placed into the medial portal. For evaluation and surgery of the lateral sesamoid, the arthroscope is placed through the dorsomedial portal and the instruments are placed into the dorsolateral portal. To evaluate the sesamoid compartment, it is helpful to release the toe traction and place the great toe into plantar flexion.

Postoperative care

Direct weight bearing is avoided for 5–7 days to decrease inflammation. Sutures are removed at 7–10 days after surgery and the patient is started on a range–of–motion and strengthening program. A stable postoperative shoe or short CAM walker is used until resolution of postoperative swelling and pain.

Outcomes

Reports indicate 83% favorable results when this technique is used for various types of pathology. The few available reports in the literature indicate favorable outcome with the procedure.[1–3]

Arthroscopy of the great toe is considered an advanced arthroscopic technique and should only be undertaken by experienced arthroscopic surgeons.

SUBTALAR JOINT ARTHROSCOPY
Indications

Indications for subtalar arthroscopy include: chondromalacia, subtalar impingement lesions, osteophytes, lysis of adhesions with posttraumatic arthrofibrosis, synovectomy, and the removal of loose bodies. Other therapeutic indications include: instability, debridement and treatment of osteochondral lesions, retrograde drilling of cystic lesions, evaluation of coalition, removal of a symptomatic os trigonum, evaluation and excision of fractures of the anterior process of the calcaneus and lateral process of the talus, and subtalar fusion.[4–20]

Contraindications

Contraindications to subtalar arthroscopy include infection and advanced degenerative joint disease with deformity. Relative contraindications include severe edema, poor vascularity, and poor skin quality.

Subtalar Joint Anatomy

For arthroscopic purposes, the subtalar joint is divided into anterior (talocalcaneonavicular) and posterior (talocalcaneal) articulations (**Fig. 7**).[21–26] The anterior and posterior articulations are separated by the tarsal canal, which has a large lateral opening called the sinus tarsi. Within the tarsal canal and sinus tarsi, the interosseous talocalcaneal ligament, the medial and intermediate roots of the inferior extensor retinaculum, the cervical ligament, fatty tissue, and blood vessels are found. The lateral ligamentous support of the subtalar joint consists of the lateral talocalcaneal ligament,

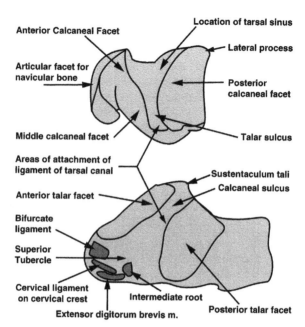

Fig. 7. Anatomy of the subtalar joint. (*From* Frey C, Di Giovanni C. Gross and arthroscopic anatomy of the foot. In: Guhl JF, Parisien JS, Boynton MD, editors. Foot and ankle arthroscopy. Third edition. New York: Springer-Verlag; 2004; with permission.)

the posterior talocalcaneal ligament, the lateral root of the inferior extensor retinaculum, and the calcaneofibular ligament (**Fig. 8**A, B).

The anterior subtalar joint is generally thought to be inaccessible to arthroscopic visualization because of the thick interosseous ligament that fills the tarsal canal. Because of this, the region normally has no connection with the posterior joint complex.

The posterior subtalar joint has a synovial lining. This joint has a posterior capsular pouch with small lateral, medial, and anterior recesses.

Examination

Motion of the subtalar joint is not simple inversion and eversion. However, motion is best tested by holding the left heel in the right hand and vice versa, then using the opposite hand to hold the forefoot and move the foot from inversion to eversion. This motion should be smooth and painless. There may be swelling or stiffness in the joint. However, although subtalar stiffness and pain may indicate pathology in and around the subtalar joint, it is not specific to one diagnosis.

Relief of symptoms with injection of local anesthetic directly into the sinus tarsi confirms the diagnosis of pain or dysfunction in the sinus tarsi (**Fig. 9**). Differential injections may be required to confirm pathology in the subtalar joint and differentiate it from ankle pathology.

Anteroposterior, lateral, and modified anteroposterior views of the foot are necessary to identify the subtalar joint. The lateral and posterior processes are better seen on hindfoot oblique views. The oblique 45-degree foot radiographs best show the anterior portion of the subtalar joint.

Broden's view shows the posterior facet of the subtalar joint. This view is obtained by rotating the foot medially 45 degrees with dorsiflexion. The x-ray beam is pointed at

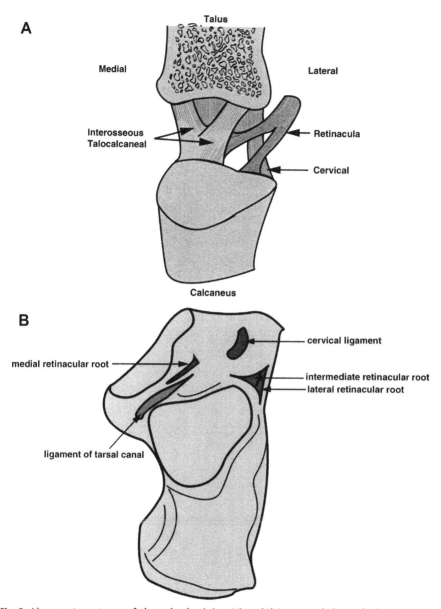

Fig. 8. Ligament anatomy of the subtalar joint. View (A) is coronal through the sinus tarsi and viewed from posterior. View (B) is the superior view of the calcaneus and sinus tarsi. (*From* Frey C, Di Giovanni C. Gross and arthroscopic anatomy of the foot. In: Guhl JF, Parisien JS, Boynton MD, editors. Foot and ankle arthroscopy. Third edition. New York: Springer-Verlag; 2004; with permission.)

the lateral malleolus and angled 10 degrees cephalad. Different views are obtained by changing the angle of the x-ray beam from 10–40 degrees (**Fig. 10**).

CT scans in the coronal plane are best for visualizing the talar body or posterior and lateral process of the talus. CT scans in the transverse or sagittal planes are best to visualize the talar neck and dome. CT can also be used to show intraarticular pathology.

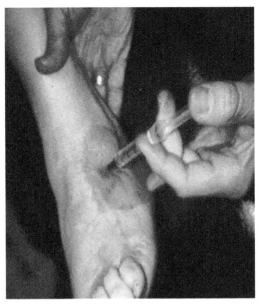

Fig. 9. Relief of symptoms with injection of local anesthetic directly into the sinus tarsi confirms the diagnosis of pain of dysfunction in the sinus tarsi.

MRI may detect chronic inflammation or fibrosis within the subtalar joint. Ligament injury, bone contusions, osteochondral lesions, chondral injury, impingement, synovitis and fibrous or cartilagenous coalitions can be well demonstrated on MRI (**Fig. 11**).

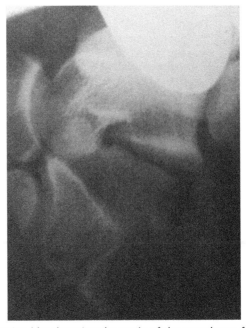

Fig. 10. Views are obtained by changing the angle of the x-ray beam from 10–40 degrees.

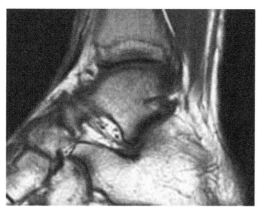

Fig. 11. Sagittal view of the subtalar joint using MRI. The cervical ligament is viewed in the sinus tarsi.

Treatment Options

Nonoperative treatment of subtalar pathology can include: injection of anesthetic agent or corticosteroids, a foot orthosis such as a UCBL, antiinflammatory medication, an ankle brace with a hindfoot lock, and peroneal tendon strengthening. Should nonoperative treatment fail, arthroscopic surgery of the subtalar joint is an option.

Equipment

2.7-mm, 30-degree short arthroscope
Small joint shaver set with a 2.0-mm and 2.9-mm shaver blade and small abrader
Arthroscopic pump
Distraction is obtained using normal saline and a gravity system
18-gauge spinal needle
High-flow system
Radiofrequency wand
Beanbag for positioning

Technique

Lateral approach

Three standard portals are recommended for visualization and instrumentation of the subtalar joint.[4] The anatomic landmarks for lateral portal placement are the lateral malleolus, the sinus tarsi, and the Achilles tendon. The anterior portal is established approximately 1 cm distal to the fibular tip and 2 cm anterior to it (**Fig. 12**). The middle portal is just anterior to the tip of the fibula, directly over the sinus tarsi. The posterior portal is at or approximately one finger width proximal to the fibular tip and 2 cm posterior to the lateral malleolus. Careful dissection and portal placement help avoid the superficial peroneal nerve branches with placement of the anterior portal and the sural nerve and peroneal tendons with placement of the posterior portal.

Surgical technique

Local, general, spinal, or epidural anesthesia can be used for this procedure. The patient is placed in the lateral decubitus position with the operative extremity draped

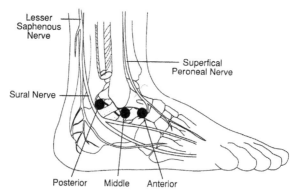

Fig. 12. Standard portals for lateral subtalar arthroscopy. (*From* Frey C, Di Giovanni C. Gross and arthroscopic anatomy of the foot. In: Guhl JF, Parisien JS, Boynton MD, editors. Foot and ankle arthroscopy. Third edition. New York: Springer-Verlag; 2004; with permission.)

free (**Fig. 13**). Padding is placed between the lower extremities,and under the contralateral extremity to protect the peroneal nerve. A tourniquet is recommended.

The anterior portal is identified first with an 18-gauge spinal needle, and the joint is inflated with a 20-cm³ syringe. A small skin incision is made and the subcutaneous tissue is gently spread using a straight mosquito clamp. A cannula with a semiblunt trochar is then placed, followed by a 2.7-mm, 30-degree oblique arthroscope. The middle portal is placed under direct visualization using an 18-gauge spinal needle and outside-in technique. The posterior portal can be placed at this time using the same direct visualization technique. The trochar is placed in an upward and slightly anterior manner. The portal is usually safe when placed behind the saphenous vein and sural nerve and anterior to the Achilles tendon. With placement of the posterior portal, care must be taken to avoid the sural nerve.

The best portal combination for access to the posterior joint is placement of the arthroscope through the anterior portal and instrumentation through the posterior portal. This allows direct visualization and access of nearly the entire surface of the posterior facet, posterior aspect of the ligaments in the sinus tarsi, the lateral capsule, and its small recess, Stieda's process (os trigonum), and the posterior pouch of the posterior joint with its synovial lining.[5,6]

The structures in the sinus tarsi, the anterior process of the calcaneus, and, occasionally, the anterior joint can be visualized best by placing the arthroscope through

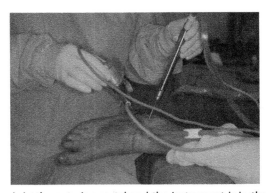

Fig. 13. Arthroscope is in the anterior portal and the instrument is in the middle portal.

the anterior portal and instrumentation through the middle portal. This portal combination is recommended for visualization and instrumentation of the sinus tarsi and anterior aspects of the posterior subtalar joint. If the ligaments that insert on the floor of the sinus tarsi are torn, damaged, or need debridement, the anterior joint can be visualized and accessed with this portal combination. Furthermore, this portal combination allows excellent visualization and access to the anterior process of the calcaneus.

The lateral approach to the subtalar joint allows direct visualization and access of the sinus tarsi, anterior process of the calcaneus, the anterior joint, the cervical ligament, practically the entire surface of the posterior facet, posterior aspect of the ligaments, the lateral capsule, and its small recess, os trigonum, and the posterior pouch of the posterior joint with its synovial lining.

Diagnostic subtalar arthroscopy examination begins with the arthroscope viewing from the anterior portal. With the arthroscope in the anterior portal (**Fig. 13**), the ligaments that insert on the floor of the sinus tarsi are visualized. It is easy to get disoriented, as the ligaments are closely packed and cross over one another in the sinus tarsi. More medially, the deep interosseous ligament (**Fig. 14**) is observed to fill the tarsal canal. The arthroscope should be now slowly withdrawn and the arthroscopic lens rotated to view the anterior joint (**Fig. 15**A, B) and the anterior process of the calcaneus (**Fig. 16**). The arthroscopic lens is then rotated in the opposite direction to view the anterior aspect of the posterior talocalcaneal articulation (**Fig. 17**). Next, the anterolateral corner of the posterior joint is examined and reflections of the lateral talocalcaneal ligament and the calcaneofibular ligament are observed (**Fig. 18**). The lateral talocalcaneal ligament is noted anterior to the calcaneofibular ligament. The arthroscopic lens may then be rotated medially and the central articulation is observed between the talus and the calcaneus. The posterolateral gutter may be seen from the anterior portal. It is often possible to advance the scope along the lateral and posterior lateral gutter and visualize the posterior pouch and Stieda's process (or os trigonum) (**Fig. 19**). The arthroscope is then switched to the posterior portal. From this view, the interosseous ligament may be seen interiorly in the joint. As the arthroscopic lens is rotated laterally, the lateral talocalcaneal ligament and calcaneofibular ligament reflections again may be seen. The central talocalcaneal joint may then be seen from this posterior view and the posterolateral gutter examined (**Fig. 20**). The posterolateral recess, posterior gutter and posterolateral corner of the talus is visualized (**Fig. 21**). The posteromedial recess and posteromedial corner of the talocalcaneal joint can be seen from the posterior portal (**Fig. 22**).

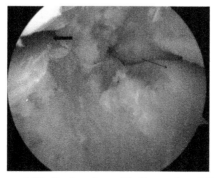

Fig. 14. Interosseous ligament fills the tarsal canal in the center of the picture. The posterior joint is to the left (*thick arrow*) and the anterior to the right (*thin arrow*).

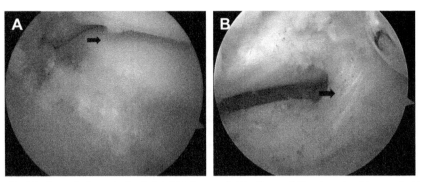

Fig. 15. (A) View of the anterior joint (*thick arrow*). The floor of the sinus tarsi is seen to the left of the joint. (B) The anterior joint of the subtalar joint. The cervical ligament is seen to the right (*black arrow*).

Posterior approach

Posterior subtalar arthroscopy can be performed using a posterolateral and postero-medial portal (**Fig. 23**).[4,14,18] This two-portal endoscopic approach to the hindfoot with the patient in the prone position provides better access to the medial and lateral aspects of the posterior subtalar joint. The main difference between the two tech-niques is that the lateral approach for subtalar arthroscopy is a true arthroscopy tech-nique in which the arthroscope and the instruments are placed within the joint while the two-portal posterior technique (using a posterolateral and posteromedial portal) starts as an extraarticular approach.

With the two-portal posterior technique, first, a working space is created adjacent to the posterior subtalar joint by removing the fatty tissue overlying the joint capsule and the posterior part of the ankle joint. The joint capsule is then partially removed to be able to inspect the joint from outside-in with the arthroscope positioned at the edge of the joint without actually entering the joint space. The maximum size of the intraar-ticular instruments depends on the available joint space.

The two-portal endoscopic approach to the hindfoot uses the posterolateral and posteromedial portals adjacent to the Achilles tendon and is performed with the

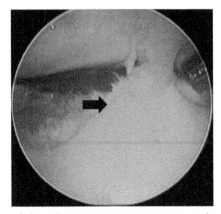

Fig. 16. Anterior process of the calcaneus. A resector is seen at the tip of the process. The floor of the sinus tarsi is to the left.

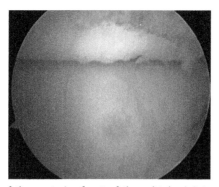

Fig. 17. Anterior aspect of the posterior facet of the subtalar joint.

patient in the prone position. The posterolateral portal is made at the level or slightly above the tip of the lateral malleolus, just lateral to the Achilles tendon. After making a vertical stab incision, the subcutaneous layer is gently split by a mosquito clamp. The mosquito clamp is directed interiorly, pointing in the direction of the interdigital web space between the first and second toe. When the tip of the clamp touches bone, it is exchanged for a 4.0-mm arthroscope sleeve with a blunt trochar. The level of the posterior subtalar joint can be determined by palpating the prominent postero-lateral talar process in the sagittal plane. The posteromedial portal is made just medial to the Achilles tendon. In the horizontal plane, it is located at the same level as the posterolateral portal. After making the skin incision, a mosquito clamp is introduced and directed toward the arthroscope shaft. When the mosquito clamp touches the shaft of the arthroscope, the shaft is used as a guide to follow anterior in the direction of the posterior subtalar joint. The mosquito clamp must touch the arthroscope shaft the entire way until the bone is reached. The blunt trochar is then exchanged for a 4.0-mm, 30-degree arthroscope. The direction of view is to the lateral side, to prevent damage to the lens system. The arthroscope is pulled slightly backward until the tip of the mosquito clamp comes into view. A clamp is used to spread the extra-articular soft tissue in front of the arthroscope tip. The mosquito clamp can now be exchanged for a 4.5-mm, full-radius resector and the posterolateral subtalar joint capsule is removed to allow visualization of the joint.

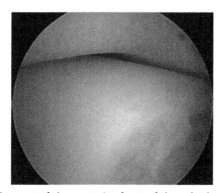

Fig. 18. Anterior lateral aspect of the posterior facet of the subtalar joint.

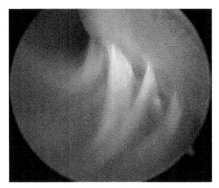

Fig. 19. Insertion of the lateral capsule of the subtalar joint onto the calcaneus.

Next, the posterior talocalcaneal ligament is debrided or penetrated to visualize the posterior and posteromedial part of the subtalar joint. In most cases, the 4.0-mm arthroscope is too large to introduce into the posterior subtalar joint. However, the posterior subtalar joint can be adequately visualized from its margins without actually entering the joint with the 4.0-mm arthroscope. Looking from outside-in, intraarticular joint pathology can be treated under direct view using the small joint instrument (**Figs. 24–26**).

Postoperative care
After completing the procedure, the portals are closed with sutures. A compression dressing is applied from the toes to the midcalf. Ice and elevation are recommended until the inflammatory phase has passed. The patient is allowed to ambulate with the use of crutches, and weight-bearing is permitted as tolerated. The sutures are removed approximately 10 days after the procedure. The patient should begin gentle active range-of-motion exercises of the foot and ankle immediately after surgery. Once the sutures are removed, if indicated, the patient is referred to a physical therapist for supervised rehabilitation. The patient should be able to return to full activities at 6–12 weeks postoperatively.

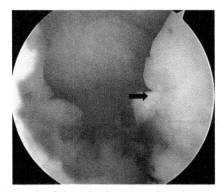

Fig. 20. Posterior lateral pouch of the subtalar joint. The calcaneus is on the right (*arrow*). The capsule is to the left.

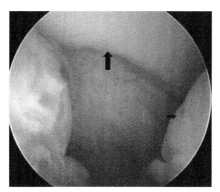

Fig. 21. Posterior pouch of the subtalar joint. The talus is on the superior aspect (*large arrow*). The calcaneus is to the right (*small arrow*).

Subtalar arthroscopy technical tips

Sinus tarsi pathology The best portal combination for the evaluation and debridement of pathology in the sinus tarsi is the arthroscope in the anterior portal and the instruments placed in the middle portal. One can debride torn interosseous ligaments, synovitis, remove loose bodies, and perform lysis of adhesions. A radiofrequency wand is a useful tool to debride the hard–to–reach spots in the sinus tarsi and subtalar joint.

Os trigonum pathology The best portal combination for evaluation and removal of the os trigonum is the arthroscope in the anterior portal and the instrumentation in the posterior portal. The os trigonum or a symptomatic Stieda's process can be debrided with a burr or shaver and removed through an arthroscopic portal using a standard arthroscopic grabber (**Fig. 27**A, B). Rarely, it is necessary to enlarge the portal for delivery of the os trigonum.

Arthroscopic subtalar arthrodesis Both the anterior and posterior portals are used in an alternating fashion during the procedure for viewing and for instrumentation. It is important to obtain a fusion of the posterior facet. The anterior facet is generally not fused. A primary synovectomy and debridement are necessary for visualization. Debridement and complete removal of the articular surface of the posterior facet of the subtalar joint down to subchondral bone is the next phase of the procedure. Once the articular cartilage has been resected, approximately 1 to 2 mm of

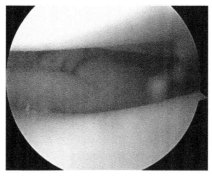

Fig. 22. View of the posterior medial recess from the posterior portal. The calcaneus is inferior and the talus is superior.

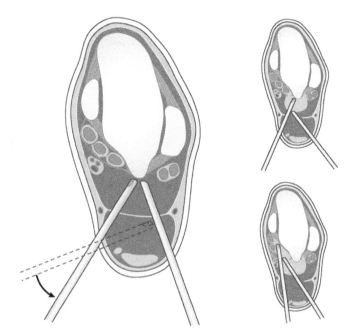

Fig. 23. Cross-section of the ankle joint at the level of the arthroscope. Arthroscope placed through the posterolateral portal, pointing in the direction of the webspace between first and second toe and a full-radius resector introduced through the posteromedial portal until it touches the arthroscope shaft. The resector glides in an anterior direction until it touches bone. (*From* Van Dijk CN, Scholten PE, Krips R. A 2-portal endoscopic approach for diagnosis and treatment of posterior ankle pathology. Arthroscopy 2000;16(8):873; with permission.)

subchondral bone is removed to expose bleeding cancellous bone. Spot-weld holes measuring approximately 2 mm deep are created on the surfaces of the calcaneus and talus to create vascular channels. The posteromedial corner is inspected to insure adequate debridement. In general, no autogenous bone graft or bone substitute is needed. The guide wire for a large cannulated screw (6.5–7mm) can be visualized as it enters the posterior facet. The foot is then put in position (about 0 to 5 degrees

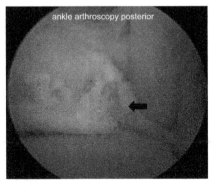

Fig. 24. View of Stieda's process (after debridement) in the foreground (*arrow*). (*From* Frey C, Di Giovanni C. Gross and arthroscopic anatomy of the foot. In: Guhl JF, Parisien JS, Boynton MD, editors. Foot and ankle arthroscopy. Third edition. New York: Springer-Verlag; 2004; with permission.)

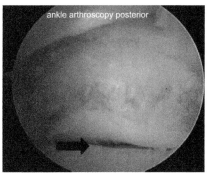

Fig. 25. Posterior arthroscopy of the subtalar joint. View of the posterior aspect of the posterior facet (*arrow*). (*From* Frey C, Di Giovanni C. Gross and arthroscopic anatomy of the foot. In: Guhl JF, Parisien JS, Boynton MD, editors. Foot and ankle arthroscopy. Third edition. New York: Springer-Verlag; 2004; with permission.)

of valgus), the guide wire advanced, followed by placement of the screw. Screw position and length is confirmed with fluoroscopy. Postoperative care is similar to open techniques.[13,15–17]

Complications

Although rare, the most likely complication to occur after subtalar arthroscopy is injury to any of the neurovascular structures in the proximity of the portals, including the sural nerve and superficial peroneal nerve. Other possible complications following subtalar joint arthroscopy include infection, instrument breakage, and damage to the articular cartilage.

Outcomes

Compared with open techniques, arthroscopy of the subtalar joint has advantages for the patient, including a faster postoperative recovery period, decreased postoperative pain and fewer complications.

Frey[9] demonstrated a success rate of 94% good-to-excellent results in the treatment of various types of subtalar pathology using arthroscopic techniques. Of the

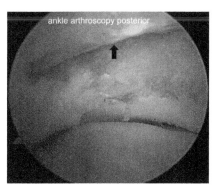

Fig. 26. Posterior arthroscopy of the subtalar joint. View of the posterior aspect of the posterior facet after debridement of capsule. The superior aspect of the posterior tibial fibular ligament is seen superiorly (*arrow*). (*From* Frey C, Di Giovanni C. Gross and arthroscopic anatomy of the foot. In: Guhl JF, Parisien JS, Boynton MD, editors. Foot and ankle arthroscopy. Third edition. New York: Springer-Verlag; 2004; with permission.)

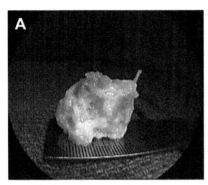 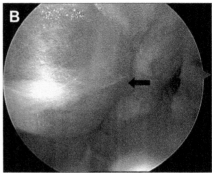

Fig. 27. (*A*) The os trigonum has been removed. (*B*) After removal of os trigonum, the flexor hallucis longus is inspected. Here, the muscle belly is seen to the left (*arrow*), with the patient's foot in dorsiflexion.

14 subjects who had a preoperative diagnosis of sinus tarsi syndrome, all the diagnoses were changed at the time of arthroscopy. The most common finding in these cases was a tear of the interosseous ligaments. In a more recent study of 126 cases, followed for over 2 years, there was a significant improvement noted using both the AOFAS and Karlsson Score.

Wiilliams and Ferkel[19] reported on the 32 months (average) follow-up of 50 subjects with hindfoot pain who underwent simultaneous ankle and subtalar arthroscopy. Preoperative diagnoses included degenerative joint disease, sinus tarsi dysfunction, and os trigonum. Good-to-excellent results were noted in 86% of the subjects. Overall, less favorable results were noted with associated ankle pathology, degenerative joint disease, increased age, and activity level of the subject. No operative complications were reported.

Goldberger and Conti[10] retrospectively reviewed 12 subjects who underwent subtalar arthroscopy for symptomatic subtalar pathology with nonspecific radiographic findings. The preoperative diagnoses were subtalar chondrosis in nine subjects and subtalar synovitis in three subjects. At 17.5 months (average) follow-up, the postoperative AOFAS hindfoot score was 71 (range 51–85) compared with a preoperative score of 66 (range, 54–79). All subjects stated that they would have the surgery again.

HAGLUND'S DEFORMITY

Indications include a painful bone prominence in the retrocalcaneal region of the posterior calcaneus in a patient who has had no relief with 6 months of conservative treatment. Contraindications include patients who have infection, open wounds, blisters, and a dysvascular extremity. Also avoid surgery on the patient who has minimum symptoms and wants a cosmetic improvement.[25–28]

Anatomy

The retrocalcaneal bursa is a consistently present, horseshoe-shaped structure that sits atop the posterior–superior aspect of the calcaneus (**Fig. 28**). The normal bursa has a volume of 1–1.5 mL. The average length of the legs is 22 mm, measured from the most superior aspect of the bursa to the most inferior aspect of the bursa legs. The average width of the legs is 4 mm and the average width of the body is 8 mm. The entire bursa has an average thickness of 4 mm, as measured from side to side.

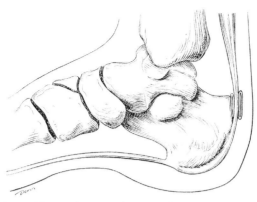

Fig. 28. The retrocalcaneal bursa sits atop the posterior–superior aspect of the calcaneus. (*From* Frey C. Calcaneal prominence resection. In: Johnson K, editor. Master Techniques in Orthopedic Surgery. Philadelphia: Lippincott Williams and Wilkins, 2002; with permission.)

The Achilles tendon does not insert at the superior aspect of the calcaneus, but significantly more inferior in the apophyseal portion of the calcaneus. The Achilles tendon sweeps backward and away from the tibia to meet the inclined calcaneus obliquely and form an acute angle.

Examination

On physical examination, the patient can be placed in the prone position on the examination table. The foot should rest in the examiner's hand and the index finger and thumb are used to palpate the medial and lateral aspects of the posterior–superior tuberosity of the calcaneus.

When the bursa is inflamed, a soft mass is felt bulging on both sides of the Achilles tendon that is painful when palpated. Dorsiflexion of the foot, which compresses the bursa between the tendon and the bone, also causes pain.

On external inspection, loss of the skin lines due to distension of the retrocalcaneal bursa may be present. In severe cases, erythema and warmth may be seen. Signs of retrocalcaneal bursitis differ from insertional Achilles tendinosis, in which there is tenderness several centimeters proximal to the tendon insertion, as well as the insertion.

Imaging

Plain weight-bearing views of the foot will help rule out other causes of hindfoot pain, such as a stress fracture, chronic infection, or tumor. No radiological criterion has been absolutely reliable when used for the diagnosis of Haglund's disease and are not predictors for preoperative symptoms or postoperative outcome. Lateral roentgenograms will reveal a thin strip of fat between the Achilles tendon and the bone proximal to the insertion of the tendon. The anterior aspect of the Achilles tendon should be sharply outlined throughout its extent by the pre-Achilles fat pad (PAFP). Retrocalcaneal bursitis is indicated when shape definition of the retrocalcaneal recess is lost and the lucency of the PAFP is replaced by soft tissue density. The distended fluid-filled bursa often projects above the calcaneus and into the PAFP. Achilles tendinosis is noted by a thickening of the tendon and loss of the sharp anterior interface with the PAFP.

Erosion of the cortex of the posterior–superior aspect of the calcaneus may be noted on lateral radiographs with chronic bursitis.

On MRI, the retrocalcaneal bursa is a potential space that is most clearly demarcated when inflamed. MRI is only recommended in those cases where making a diagnosis is difficult.

Treatment Options

Nonoperative treatment includes nonsteroidal antiinflammatory medication, heel lifts, soft heel counters and a backless shoe. Running athletes should decrease mileage and stop training on hills and hard surfaces. Tight calf muscles, tight hamstrings, or a cavus foot may be associated and should be stretched. A cavus foot may require a custom orthotic device.

Most patients respond to conservative treatment in the first 6 months.

Instrumentation

- Micro sagittal saw
- Micro reciprocating rasp
- Small curette
- 2.9-mm arthroscope and small joint instrumentation
- 18-gauge spinal needle
- Straight mosquito
- Standard foot tray

Arthroscopic Technique

The retrocalcaneal space may be approached endoscopically. The patient is placed in the prone position, with a bump under the ankle. The medial and lateral borders of the Achilles tendon are palpated. The posterior superior aspect of the calcaneus is also readily located.

Medial and lateral portals are placed just above the superior aspect of the calcaneus, medial and lateral to the Achilles tendon (**Fig. 29**). Care must be taken when making the medial portal, because the calcaneal branch of the lateral plantar nerve is at risk for injury in this region. The medial portal is made under direct visualization by introducing an 18-guage spinal needle just proximal to the superior medial border of the os calcis.

A 2.9-mm arthroscope and a small joint instrumentation are used interchangeably through these portals. The arthroscope with a blunt trochar is introduced into the bursa after making a skin incision just proximal to the superior lateral border of the os calcis. A full-radius synovial shaver is used to remove the bursa.

Once the bursa is removed, a small acrominizer or abrader is used to remove the Haglund's deformity, starting at the posterior–superior aspect of the calcaneus and proceeding inferior 2–4 cm to the superior attachment site of the Achilles tendon. It is important to dorsiflexion the ankle to check for further impingement (**Fig. 30**).

The location of even a small portal in the area of the sural nerve (lateral portal) or the calcaneal branches of the lateral plantar nerve (medial portal) can cause a long period of postoperative tenderness aggravated by a firm heel counter on a shoe. To successfully decompress the retrocalcaneal space, adequate bone must be removed. Bone can be removed up to the insertion site of the Achilles tendon.

The area of calcaneal prominence is palpated repeatedly through the overlying skin to make sure that all ridges and spikes are removed. It is possible to remove too much distal bone and cut into the insertion of the Achilles tendon. This could allow the tendon to avulse later. Careful exposure of the insertion site should help avoid this pitfall.

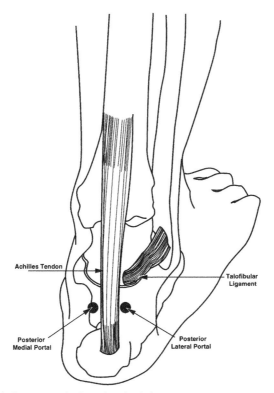

Fig. 29. The portals for removal of Haglund's deformity.

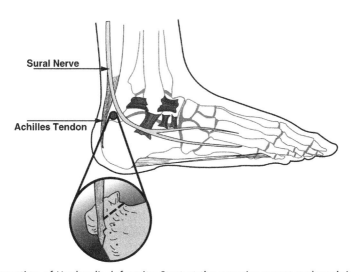

Fig. 30. Resection of Haglund's deformity. Start at the superior aspect and work inferiorly.

Postoperative Care

The patient is placed into a short-leg, non–weight-bearing cast with the foot in mild plantar flexion for the first 1–2 weeks. A short-leg walking cast with the foot gradually repositioned up to neutral is used for the next 2 weeks. When the cast is removed, the patient is placed into a shoe with a $5^7/_{16}$-in, tapered internal heel lift that is gradually reduced to $^3/_{16}$ of an inch, and this worn for 3 months. General muscle conditioning should begin when the cast is removed.

Outcomes

A review of the literature indicates that 73–97% good-to-excellent results have been reported with the open procedure.[27–30]

TENDOSCOPY
Indications

The main indication for tendoscopy is inflammatory and adhesive tenosynovitis. Ruptures, dislocations, and degenerative tendinosis may also be evaluated and debrided. In the case of peroneal tendon tendinosis, where debridement of up to 50% of the tendon may resolve patient complaints, this is an especially effective technique to use. This is considered an advanced arthroscopic technique.[30,31]

Instrumentation

2.7–2.9 mm arthroscope with 30-degree angulation
Small joint instrumentation
18-gauge spinal needle
Radiofrequency wand
Arthroscopic pump

Technique

Arthroscopic portals for access to the tendons can be obtained anywhere along the tendons. The two main portals for posterior tibial and peroneal tendoscopy are located directly over the tendon sheaths. The portals are placed approximately 1.5–2.0 cm distal and 1.5–2.0 cm proximal to the posterior edge of the lateral or medial malleolus (**Fig. 31**A). The distal portal is usually made first with an incision over the skin. An 18-gauge spinal needle is directed into the tendon sheath under direct visualization to help place the proximal portals. An incision is then made through the skin. Instrumentation can be introduced as necessary through either portal. Synovectomy is performed with a shaver or radiofrequency wand.

On the medial side, the distal portal is used for a complete inspection of the posterior tibial tendon from its insertion on the navicular bone to around 6–8 cm above the level of the medial malleolus. Once the scope is introduced, it is rotated for complete visualization.

On the lateral side, the distal portal can be used for a complete view of the peroneal tendons. The inspection can start about 6 cm proximal to the posterior tibial margin of the lateral malleolus. There is a thin membrane that splits the peroneus brevis and longus tendons into two compartments. More distally, both tendons lie in one compartment until they again split distal to the lateral malleolus. Both tendons can be inspected by rotating the arthroscope. In addition the tendons, mesotenon and tendon sheaths can be inspected.

On the lateral side, the peroneal tendon sheath may be entered while performing a lateral subtalar arthroscopy, especially if there is a tear of the lateral capsule and/

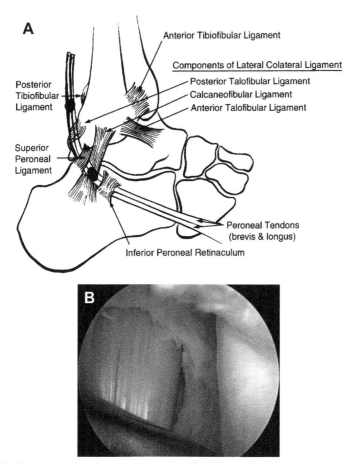

Fig. 31. (A) The portal sites for tendonoscopy of the peroneal tendons. (B) The peroneal tendons are seen through a tear of the STJ capsule.

or the calcaneofibular ligament (**Fig. 31**B). This is most commonly seen in patients who have chronic instability of the ankle or subtalar joint. Care should be taken in these patients to inspect the lateral capsule for tears and exposed peroneal tendons before aggressive debridement techniques are used (**Fig. 32**).

Postoperative Care

The wounds are closed in a standard fashion and the patient is placed into a compressive dressing with a splint. It is recommended in most cases of tenosynovitis that the patient remain non-weight bearing for 5–10 days, until the inflammatory phase has passed. The patient is then placed into a cast boot, the sutures are removed at 14 days, and gentle active range of motion is begun. Depending on the involvement of the tendon, a cast or cast boot may be used for 4–6 weeks.

SUMMARY

These arthroscopic alternatives to open procedures can be helpful for evaluating and treating common foot and ankle injuries. These techniques can also result in a shorter

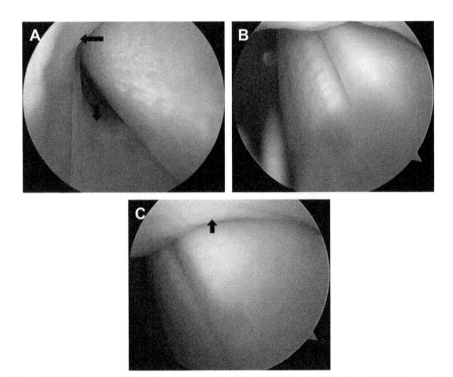

Fig. 32. (A) The peroneal tendons are seen to the right. The tendon sheath (*left arrow*) is clearly seen and free of lesions. The mesotenon is seen on the inferior aspect of this view (*down arrow*). (B) Tendoscopy of the peroneus longus and brevis tendons. (C) Tendoscopy of the peroneal tendons. The superior retinaculum is seen at the top of this view (*arrow*).

and more comfortable recovery. However, the surgeon must gain significant experience with open procedures and have a very good grasp of arthroscopic techniques in order to begin use of these advanced techniques. We look forward to developing further indications and uses of less-invasive techniques to assist the athlete and others in their recovery.

REFERENCES

1. Bartlett DH. Arthroscopic management of osteochondritis dissecans of the first metatarsal head. Arthroscopy 1988;4:51–4.
2. Frey CC, van Dijk NC. Arthroscopy of the great toe. In: James CY Chow, editor. Advanced Arthroscopy. New York: Springer–Verlag; 2001. p. 675–82.
3. Lundeen RD. Arthroscopic approaches to the joints of the foot. J Am Podiatr Med Assoc 1987;77:451–6.
4. Beimers H, Frey C, van Dijk N. Arthroscopy of the posterior subtalar joint. Foot and Ankle 2006;11:369–90.
5. Cheng JC, Ferkel RD. The role of arthroscopy in ankle and subtalar degenerative joint disease. Clin Orthop Relat Res 1998;349:65–72.
6. de Palma L, Santucci A, Ventura A, et al. Anatomy and embryology of the talocalcaneal joint. Foot Ankle Surg 2003;9:7–18.
7. Frey C, Feder K, Chow H. Arthroscopy of the subtalar joint: clinical outcomes. Submitted to Foot Ankle Int 2008;29:842–4.

8. Frey C, Gasser S, Feder K. Arthroscopy of the subtalar joint. Foot Ankle Int 1994; 15(8):424–8.

9. Frey C, Feder KS, DiGiovanni C. Arthroscopic evaluation of the subtalar joint: does sinus tarsi syndrome exist? Foot Ankle Int 1999;20(3):185–91.

10. Goldberger MI, Conti SF. Clinical outcome after subtalar arthroscopy. Foot Ankle Int 1998;19(7):462–5.

11. Parisien JS. Arthroscopy of the posterior subtalar joint. In: Parisien JS, editor. Current techniques in arthroscopy. Third Edition. New York: Thieme; 1998. p. 161–8.

12. Parisien JS. Posterior subtalar joint arthroscopy. In: Guhl JF, Parisien JS, Boynton MD, editors. Foot and ankle arthroscopy. Third Edition. New York: Springer-Verlag; 2004. p. 175–82.

13. Scranton PE Jr. Comparison of open isolated subtalar arthrodesis with autogenous bone graft versus outpatient arthroscopic subtalar arthrodesis using injectable bone morphogenic protein-enhanced graft. Foot Ankle Int 1999;20(3):162–5.

14. Sitler DF, Amendola A, Bailey CS, et al. Posterior ankle arthroscopy: an anatomic study. J Bone Joint Surg Am 2002;84(A(5)):763–9.

15. Stroud CC. Arthroscopic arthrodesis of the ankle, subtalar, and first metatarsophalangeal joint. Foot Ankle Clin 2002;7(1):135–46.

16. Tasto JP. Arthroscopic subtalar arthrodesis. In: Guhl JF, Parisien JS, Boynton MD, editors. Foot and ankle arthroscopy. Third edition. New York: Springer-Verlag; 2004. p. 183–90.

17. Tasto JP, Frey C, Laimans P, et al. Arthroscopic ankle arthrodesis. Instr Course Lect 2000;49:259–80.

18. Van Dijk CN, Scholten PE, Krips R. A 2-portal endoscopic approach for diagnosis and treatment of posterior ankle pathology. Arthroscopy 2000;16(8):871–6.

19. Williams MM, Ferkel RD. Subtalar arthroscopy: indications, technique, and results. Arthroscopy 1998;14(4):373–81.

20. Inman VT. The subtalar joint. In: Beals RK, editor. The joints of the ankle. Baltimore: Williams & Wilkins Company; 1976. p. 35–44.

21. Jaivin JS, Ferkel RD. Arthroscopy of the foot and ankle. Clin Sports Med 1994; 13(4):761–83.

22. Harper MC. The lateral ligamentous support of the subtalar joint. Foot Ankle 1991; 11(6):354–8.

23. Parisien JS. Arthroscopy of the posterior subtalar joint: a preliminary report. Foot Ankle 1986;6(5):219–24.

24. Perry J. Anatomy and biomechanics of the hindfoot. Clin Orthop 1983;177:9–15.

25. Lapidus PW. Subtalar joint, its anatomy and mechanics. Bull Hosp Joint Dis 1955; 16(2):179–95.

26. Viladot A, Lorenzo JC, Salazar J, et al. The subtalar joint: embryology and morphology. Foot Ankle 1984;5(2):54–66.

27. Sammarco G, Taylor A. Operative management of Haglund's deformity in the nonathlete: a retrospective study. Foot and Ankle International 2000;19:724–9.

28. Scholten PE, Altena MC, Krips R, et al. Treatment of a large intraosseous talar ganglion by means of hindfoot endoscopy. Arthroscopy 2003;19(1):96–100.

29. Van Dijk CN, van Dyk E, Scholten P, et al. Tendoscopic calcaneoplasty. Am J Sports Med 2001;29:185–9.

30. Van Dijk CN. Hindfoot endoscopy for posterior ankle pain. In: Guhil JF, Parisien JS, Boynton MD, editors. Foot and Ankle Arthoscopy. New York: Springer Verlag; 2004. p. 545–54.

31. Van Dijk CN, Kort N, Scholten P. Tendoscopy of the posterior tibial tendon. Arthroscopy 1997;6:692–8.

Index

Note: Page numbers of article titles are in **boldface** type.

A

Accessory navicular, navicular stress fracture vs., 194–195
Achilles tendon, arthroscopic consideration of, in Haglund's deformity, 332–335
    in insertional tendinopathy, 270–271
    in subtalar joint, 323–324, 326–327
  insertional tendinopathy of, description of, 266–267
    MRI stratification of, 267
    noninsertional vs., 260–261
    surgical treatment of, 267–271
      algorithm for, 268
      arthroscopic debridement in, 270–271
      goals for, 267–268
      Haglund's deformity and, 270–271
      lateral incision for, 270–271
      medial incision with detachment for, 269
      midline incision for, 268–269
      sports approach in, 271
    treatment of, 267–271
  rupture of, **247–275**. See also *Achilles tendon ruptures.*
  stretch exercise, for plantar heel pain, 234, 240–241
Achilles tendon complex, anatomy of, 247–248
Achilles tendon ruptures, **247–275**
  acute, definition of, 253
    management of, 249–253
  anatomy and, 247–248
  chronic, definition of, 253–254
    evaluation of, 254
    management of, 253–260
  degeneration stages and, 260–263
  evaluation of, 248–249, 254
  imaging of, 248–249, 258
  incidence of, 248
  inflammation stages and, 260–262
  management of, 249–260
    acute, 249–253
    chronic, 253–260
    immobilization indications in, 250–251, 254, 269
  nonoperative management of, acute, 250
    goals for, 249–250
    results of, 250–251

Foot Ankle Clin N Am 14 (2009) 341–368
doi:10.1016/S1083-7515(09)00053-9
1083-7515/09/$ – see front matter © 2009 Elsevier Inc. All rights reserved.
foot.theclinics.com

none

Moving?

Make sure your subscription moves with you!

To notify us of your new address, find your **Clinics Account Number** (located on your mailing label above your name), and contact customer service at:

E-mail: elspcs@elsevier.com

800-654-2452 (subscribers in the U.S. & Canada)
314-453-7041 (subscribers outside of the U.S. & Canada)

Fax number: 314-523-5170

Elsevier Periodicals Customer Service
11830 Westline Industrial Drive
St. Louis, MO 63146

*To ensure uninterrupted delivery of your subscription, please notify us at least 4 weeks in advance of move.

ELSEVIER

Printed and bound by CPI Group (UK) Ltd, Croydon, CR0 4YY

03/10/2024

01040465-0007